Use of Biologic and Regenerative Therapies in Equine Practice

Editor

LAUREN V. SCHNABEL

VETERINARY CLINICS OF NORTH AMERICA: EQUINE PRACTICE

www.vetequine.theclinics.com

Consulting Editor

RAMIRO E. TORIBIO

December 2023 • Volume 39 • Number 3

ELSEVIER

1600 John F. Kennedy Boulevard • Suite 1800 • Philadelphia, Pennsylvania, 19103-2899

http://www.vetequine.theclinics.com

VETERINARY CLINICS OF NORTH AMERICA: EQUINE PRACTICE Volume 39, Number 3
December 2023 ISSN 0749-0739, ISBN-13: 978-0-323-93891-4

Editor: Taylor Hayes
Developmental Editor: Akshay Samson

Veterinary Clinics of North America: Equine Practice (ISSN 0749-0739) is published in April, August, and December by Elsevier Inc., 360 Park Avenue South, New York, NY 10010-1710. Business and Editorial Offices: 1600 John F. Kennedy Blvd., Suite 1800, Philadelphia, PA 19103-2899. Subscription prices are $308.00 per year (domestic individuals), $647.00 per year (domestic institutions), $100.00 per year (domestic students/residents), $351.00 per year (Canadian individuals), $814.00 per year (Canadian institutions), $383.00 per year (international individuals), $814.00 per year (international institutions), $100.00 per year (Canadian students/residents), and $180.00 per year (international students/residents). To receive student/resident rate, orders must be accompanied by name of affiliated institution, date of term, and the signature of program/residency coordinator on institution letterhead. Orders will be billed at individual rate until proof of status is received. Foreign air speed delivery is included in all *Clinics* subscription prices. All prices are subject to change without notice. **POSTMASTER:** Send address changes to *Veterinary Clinics of North America: Equine Practice*, 3251 Riverport Lane, Maryland Heights, MO 63043. Customer Service (orders, claims, online, change of address): Elsevier Health Sciences Division, Subscription **Customer Service, 3251 Riverport Lane, Maryland Heights, MO 63043. Tel: 1-800-654-2452 (U.S. and Canada); 314-447-8871 (outside U.S. and Canada). Fax: 314-447-8029. E-mail: journalscustomerservice-usa@elsevier.com (for print support);** E-mail: **journalsonlinesupport-usa@elsevier.com (for online support).**

Reprints. For copies of 100 or more of articles in this publication, please contact the Commercial Reprints Department, Elsevier Inc., 360 Park Avenue South, New York, NY 10010-1710. Tel.: 212-633-3874; Fax: 212-633-3820; E-mail: reprints@elsevier.com.

Veterinary Clinics of North America: Equine Practice is covered in *MEDLINE/PubMed (Index Medicus), Excerpta Medica, Current Contents/Agriculture, Biology and Environmental Sciences, and ISI.*

Contributors

CONSULTING EDITOR

RAMIRO E. TORIBIO, DVM, MS, PhD, DACVIM
Diplomate, American College of Veterinary Internal Medicine; Professor and Trueman Endowed Chair of Equine Medicine and Surgery, College of Veterinary Medicine, The Ohio State University, Columbus, Ohio, USA

EDITOR

LAUREN V. SCHNABEL, DVM, PhD, DACVS, DACVSMR
Diplomate, American College of Veterinary Surgeons; Diplomate, American College of Veterinary Sports Medicine and Rehabilitation; Professor of Equine Orthopedic Surgery, Department of Clinical Sciences, North Carolina State University College of Veterinary Medicine, Associate Director, Comparative Medicine Institute, North Carolina State University, Raleigh, North Carolina, USA

AUTHORS

JENNIFER G. BARRETT, PhD, DVM, DACVS, DACVSMR
Diplomate, American College of Veterinary Surgeons; Diplomate, American College of Veterinary Sports Medicine and Rehabilitation; Theodora Ayer Randolph Professor of Equine Surgery, Marion duPont Scott Equine Medical Center, Virginia-Maryland College of Veterinary Medicine, Virginia Tech, Leesburg, Virginia, USA

MYRA BARRETT, DVM, MS, DACVR, DACVR-EDI
Diplomate, American College of Veterinary Radiology; Diplomate, American College of Veterinary Radiology - Equine Diagnostic Imaging; Department of Environmental and Radiological Health Sciences, College of Veterinary Medicine, Colorado State University, Fort Collins, Colorado, USA

LINDSEY BOONE, DVM, PhD, DACVS-LA
Diplomate, American College of Veterinary Surgeons - Large Animal; Associate Professor of Equine Surgery and Sports Medicine, Department of Clinical Sciences, Auburn University College of Veterinary Medicine, John Thomas Vaughan Large Animal Teaching Hospital, Auburn, Alabama, USA

LYNDAH CHOW, PhD
Research Scientist, Department of Clinical Sciences, College of Veterinary Medicine and Biomedical Sciences, Colorado State University, Fort Collins, Colorado, USA

AIMEE C. COLBATH, VMD, PhD, DACVS-LA
Diplomate, American College of Veterinary Surgeons - Large Animal; Assistant Professor of Large Animal Orthopedic Surgery, Department of Clinical Sciences, Cornell University College of Veterinary Medicine, Ithaca, New York, USA

STEVEN W. DOW, DVM, PhD, DACVIM
Diplomate, American College of Veterinary Internal Medicine; Principal Investigator, Departments of Clinical Sciences, and Microbiology, Immunology and Pathology, College of Veterinary Medicine and Biomedical Sciences, Colorado State University, Fort Collins, Colorado, USA

LISA A. FORTIER, DVM, PhD, DACVS
Diplomate, American College of Veterinary Surgeons; Clinical Sciences, Cornell University College of Veterinary Medicine, Ithaca, New York, USA

CHRISTOPHER W. FRYE, DVM, DACVSMR
Diplomate, American College of Veterinary Sports Medicine and Rehabilitation; Associate Clinical Professor of Sports Medicine and Rehabilitation, Department of Clinical Sciences, Cornell University College of Veterinary Medicine, Ithaca, New York, USA

LARRY D. GALUPPO, DVM, DACVS
Diplomate, American College of Veterinary Surgeons; Department of Surgical and Radiological Sciences, School of Veterinary Medicine, University of California, Davis, Davis, California, USA

JESSICA M. GILBERTIE, DVM, MS, PhD
Assistant Professor, Department of Microbiology and Immunology, Edward Via College of Osteopathic Medicine, Blacksburg, Virginia, USA

BRIAN CHRISTOPHER GILGER, DVM, MS, Dipl ACVO, Dipl ABT
Diplomate, American College of Veterinary Ophthalmologists; Diplomate, American Board of Toxicology; Professor of Ophthalmology, North Carolina State University, Raleigh, North Carolina, USA

LAURIE R. GOODRICH, DVM, MS, PhD, DACVS
Diplomate, American College of Veterinary Surgeons; Professor, Department of Clinical Sciences, College of Veterinary Medicine and Biomedical Sciences, Colorado State University, Fort Collins, Colorado, USA

REBECCA M. HARMAN, PhD
Baker Institute for Animal Health, College of Veterinary Medicine, Cornell University, Ithaca, New York, USA

CAITLYN R. HORNE, DVM, DACVSMR
Diplomate, American College of Veterinary Sports Medicine and Rehabilitation; North Carolina State University College of Veterinary Medicine, Raleigh, North Carolina, USA

THOMAS G. KOCH, DVM, PhD
Associate Professor, Department of Biomedical Sciences, Ontario Veterinary College, University of Guelph, Guelph, Ontario, Canada

ALEXANDER G. KUZMA-HUNT, BSc
Department of Biomedical Sciences, Ontario Veterinary College, University of Guelph, Guelph, Ontario, Canada

ELIZABETH S. MACDONALD, BVMS, MS, DACVIM
Diplomate, American College of Veterinary Internal Medicine; Clinical Instructor, Marion duPont Scott Equine Medical Center, Virginia-Maryland College of Veterinary Medicine, Virginia Tech, Leesburg, Virginia, USA

TARALYN M. MCCARREL, DVM, DACVS-LA
Diplomate, American College of Veterinary Surgeons - Large Animal; Clinical Assistant Professor, Department of Large Animal Clinical Sciences, University of Florida College of Veterinary Medicine, Gainesville, Florida, USA

KYLA F. ORTVED, DVM, PhD, DACVS, DACVSMR
Diplomate, American College of Veterinary Surgeons; Diplomate, American College of Veterinary Sports Medicine and Rehabilitation; Associate Professor of Large Animal Surgery, Jacques Jenny Endowed Chair of Orthopedic Surgery, Clinical Studies-New Bolton Center, University of Pennsylvania, Kennett Square, Pennsylvania, USA

JOHN PERONI, DVM, MS, DACVS
Diplomate, American College of Veterinary Surgeons; Dr. Steeve Giguere Memorial Professor in Large Animal Medicine, Department of Large Animal Medicine, University of Georgia College of Veterinary Medicine, Athens, Georgia, USA

LYNN M. PEZZANITE, DVM, MS, PhD, DACVS-LA
Diplomate, American College of Veterinary Surgeons - Large Animal; Assistant Professor, Department of Clinical Sciences, College of Veterinary Medicine and Biomedical Sciences, Colorado State University, Fort Collins, Colorado, USA

AARTHI RAJESH, PhD
Baker Institute for Animal Health, College of Veterinary Medicine, Cornell University, Ithaca, New York, USA

KEITH A. RUSSELL, PhD
Department of Biomedical Sciences, Ontario Veterinary College, University of Guelph, Guelph, Ontario, Canada

LAUREN V. SCHNABEL, DVM, PhD, DACVS, DACVSMR
Diplomate, American College of Veterinary Surgeons; Diplomate, American College of Veterinary Sports Medicine and Rehabilitation; Professor of Equine Orthopedic Surgery, Department of Clinical Sciences, North Carolina State University College of Veterinary Medicine, Associate Director, Comparative Medicine Institute, North Carolina State University, Raleigh, North Carolina, USA

MATHIEU SPRIET, DVM, MS, DACVR, DECVDI, DACVR-EDI
Diplomate, American College of Veterinary Radiology; Diplomate, European College of Veterinary Diagnostic Imaging; Diplomate, American College of Veterinary Radiology - Equine Diagnostic Imaging; Department of Surgical and Radiological Sciences, School of Veterinary Medicine, University of California, Davis, Davis, California, USA

SARA TUFTS, DVM
Resident, North Carolina State University College of Veterinary Medicine, Raleigh, North Carolina, USA

GERLINDE R. VAN DE WALLE, DVM, PhD
Associate Professor, Department of Microbiology and Immunology, Baker Institute for Animal Health, College of Veterinary Medicine, Cornell University, Ithaca, New York, USA

BETSY VAUGHAN, DVM, DACVSMR
Diplomate, American College of Sports Medicine and Rehabilitation; Department of Surgical and Radiological Sciences, School of Veterinary Medicine, University of California, Davis, Davis, California, USA

ASHLEE E. WATTS, DVM, PhD, DACVS
Diplomate, American College of Veterinary Surgeons; College Station, Texas, USA

TARALYN M. MCCARREL, DVM, DACVS-LA
Diplomate, American College of Veterinary Surgeons - Large Animal; Clinical Assistant Professor, Department of Large Animal Clinical Sciences, University of Florida College of Veterinary Medicine, Gainesville, Florida, USA

KYLA F. ORTVED, DVM, PhD, DACVS, DACVSMR
Diplomate, American College of Veterinary Surgeons; Diplomate, American College of Veterinary Sports Medicine and Rehabilitation; Associate Professor of Large Animal Surgery, Jacques Jenny Endowed Chair of Orthopedic Surgery, Clinical Studies New Bolton Center, University of Pennsylvania, Kennett Square, Pennsylvania, USA

JOHN PERONI, DVM, MS, DACVS
Diplomate, American College of Veterinary Surgeons; Dr. Steeve Giguère Memorial Professor in Large Animal Medicine, Department of Large Animal Medicine, University of Georgia College of Veterinary Medicine, Athens, Georgia, USA

LYNN M. PEZZANITE, DVM, MS, PhD, DACVS-LA
Diplomate, American College of Veterinary Surgeons - Large Animal; Assistant Professor, Department of Clinical Sciences, College of Veterinary Medicine and Biomedical Sciences, Colorado State University, Fort Collins, Colorado, USA

KARTHIK RAJESH, PhD
Baker Institute for Animal Health, College of Veterinary Medicine, Cornell University, Ithaca, New York, USA

KEITH A. RUSSELL, PhD
Department of Biomedical Sciences, Ontario Veterinary College, University of Guelph, Guelph, Ontario, Canada

LAUREN V. SCHNABEL, DVM, PhD, DACVS, DACVSMR
Diplomate, American College of Veterinary Surgeons; Diplomate, American College of Veterinary Sports Medicine and Rehabilitation; Professor of Equine Orthopedic Surgery, Department of Clinical Sciences, North Carolina State University College of Veterinary Medicine; Associate Director, Comparative Medicine Institute, North Carolina State University, Raleigh, North Carolina, USA

MATHIEU SPRIET, DVM, MS, DACVR, DECVDI, DACVR-EDI
Diplomate, American College of Veterinary Radiology; Diplomate, European College of Veterinary Diagnostic Imaging; Diplomate, American College of Veterinary Radiology's Equine Diagnostic Imaging, Department of Surgical and Radiological Sciences, School of Veterinary Medicine, University of California, Davis, Davis, California, USA

SARA TUFTS, DVM
Resident, North Carolina State University College of Veterinary Medicine, Raleigh, North Carolina, USA

GERLINDE R. VAN DE WALLE, DVM, PhD
Associate Professor, Department of Microbiology and Immunology, Baker Institute for Animal Health, College of Veterinary Medicine, Cornell University, Ithaca, New York, USA

BETSY VAUGHAN, DVM, DACVSMR
Diplomate, American College of Sports Medicine and Rehabilitation; Department of Surgical and Radiological Sciences, School of Veterinary Medicine, University of California, Davis, Davis, California, USA

ASHLEE E. WATTS, DVM, PhD, DACVS
Diplomate, American College of Veterinary Surgeons; College Station, Texas, USA

Contents

Preface: Considerations for the Use of Biologic and Regenerative Therapies in Equine Practice xiii

Lauren V. Schnabel

Dedications xv

Introduction to Equine Biologic and Regenerative Therapies 419

Lindsey Boone and John Peroni

Regenerative medicine is defined as the process of replacing or regenerating cells, tissues, or organs to restore or establish normal function. The use of regenerative medicine in equine practice to treat injured musculoskeletal tissues with limited capacity for intrinsic healing is growing. This article provides the practitioner with a brief and basic overview of the regenerative products currently used in equine practice.

Equine Platelet-Rich Plasma 429

Taralyn M. McCarrel

Platelet-rich plasma (PRP) is an orthobiologic therapy composed of platelets, leukocytes, red blood cells, and plasma proteins. PRP has been used for 20 years, but progress determining efficacy has been slow. The definitions and classification of PRP are reviewed, and the use of PRP for tendon, ligament, and joint disease is discussed with a focus on findings of basic science and clinical studies, platelet activation, concurrent administration of nonsteroidal anti-inflammatory drugs, and treatment complications. Finally, the advantages of platelet lysates and freeze-dried platelets are discussed. The promising results of a PRP lysate optimized for antibiofilm and antimicrobial properties are introduced.

Equine Autologous Conditioned Serum and Autologous Protein Solution 443

Kyla F. Ortved

Orthobiologics are used with increasing frequency in equine musculoskeletal disease to improve the quality of the repair tissue and prevent reinjury. Autologous blood-based products, or hemoderivatives, are made by processing the patient's blood using different systems to produce a final therapeutic product. Autologous conditioned serum (ACS) and autologous protein solution (APS) are commonly used to treat joint disorders and can also be used treat tendon and ligament injuries. Hemoderivatives contain increased concentrations of anti-inflammatory and immunomodulatory cytokines, and growth factors that help direct tissue healing and repair. The specifics of ACS and APS for treatment of musculoskeletal injuries are discussed.

Equine Bone Marrow Aspirate Concentrate 453

Lisa A. Fortier

Bone marrow concentrate is generated by centrifugation of bone marrow aspirate. It contains mesenchymal stromal cells, anabolic chemokines/cytokines, and supraphysiological concentrations of interleukin-1 receptor antagonist protein (IL-1RA). It is an effective treatment for osteoarthritis or desmitis, or as an adjunct in surgery to enhance bone or cartilage repair.

Overview of Equine Stem Cells: Sources, Practices, and Potential Safety Concerns 461

Thomas G. Koch, Alexander G. Kuzma-Hunt, and Keith A. Russell

Over the past 2 decades, equine veterinarians are turning increasingly to stem cell therapies to repair damaged tissues or to promote healing through modulation of the immune system. Research is ongoing into optimizing practices associated with stem cell product transport, dosage, and administration. Culture-expanded equine mesenchymal stem cell therapies seem safe, even when used allogeneically, but various safety concerns should be considered. Stem cells and cellular reprogramming tools hold great promise for future equine therapies.

Use of Stem Cells for the Treatment of Musculoskeletal Injuries in Horses 475

Ashlee E. Watts

Mesenchymal stem cells (MSCs) are used as a regenerative therapy in horses for musculoskeletal injury since the late 1990s and in some regions are standard of care for certain injuries. Yet, there is no Food and Drug Administration–approved MSC therapeutic in the United States for horses. In humans, lack of regulatory approval in the United States has been caused by failure of late-phase clinical trials to demonstrate consistent efficacy, perhaps because of nonuniformity of MSC preparation and application techniques. This article discusses clinical evidence for musculoskeletal applications of MSCs in the horse and current challenges to marketing approval.

Advances in Imaging Techniques to Guide Therapies and Monitor Response to the Treatment of Musculoskeletal Injuries 489

Caitlyn R. Horne and Sara Tufts

Continual advancements in diagnostic imaging have allowed for more accurate and complete diagnoses of injuries in the performance horse. The use of several different imaging tools has further allowed the equine sports medicine clinician to more carefully direct treatment options, monitor response to therapy and guide rehabilitation recommendations. The advancements in diagnostic imaging and novel treatment options have led to the improvement in the overall prognosis of many injuries that affect the horse and their performance. The purpose of this section is to review the advancements made in diagnostic imaging of the horse and to aid the practitioner in the selection of the appropriate modality and how best to use them to guide treatment and monitoring decisions.

Advances in Regional Vascular Injection Techniques for the Delivery of Stem Cells to Musculoskeletal Injury Sites **503**

Mathieu Spriet, Betsy Vaughan, Myra Barrett, and Larry D. Galuppo

Vascular injections of stem cells are a pertinent alternative to direct intralesional injections when treating multiple or extensive lesions or with lesions impossible to reach directly. Extensive research using stem cell tracking has shown that intra-arterial injections without the use of a tourniquet should be preferred over venous or arterial regional limb perfusion techniques using a tourniquet. The median artery is used for the front limbs and the cranial tibial artery for the hind limbs. Proper efficacy studies are still lacking but early clinical work seems promising.

Interactions Between Biologic Therapies and Other Treatment Modalities **515**

Aimee C. Colbath and Christopher W. Frye

Biologic therapies are becoming increasingly utilized by veterinarians. The literature regarding the interaction of biologic therapies with other therapeutics is still in its infancy. Initial studies have examined the effects of exercise, stress, various pharmaceutical interventions, extracorporeal shockwave, therapeutic laser, and hyperbaric oxygen on biologic therapies. Continued research is imperative as owners and veterinarians increasingly choose a multimodal approach to injury and illness. Further, understanding the effects of concurrently administered treatments and pharmaceuticals as well as the health status of the horse is imperative to providing the optimal therapeutic outcome.

Use of Biologics and Stem Cells for Wound Healing in the Horse **525**

Rebecca M. Harman, Aarthi Rajesh, and Gerlinde R. Van de Walle

Treatment of skin wounds is a high priority in veterinary medicine because healthy uncompromised skin is essential for the well-being of horses. Stem cells and other biologic therapies offer benefits by reducing the need for surgical procedures and conventional antibiotics. Evidence from in vitro studies and small in vivo trials supports the use of equine stem cells and biologics for the treatment of acute and chronic cutaneous wounds. Larger clinical trials are warranted to better evaluate the regenerative and immunological responses to these treatments. Additionally, delivery methods and treatment schedules should be optimized to improve efficacy of these novel therapies.

Use of Biologics and Stem Cells in Equine Ophthalmology **541**

Brian Christopher Gilger

Regenerative therapy and biologics have the promise to treat equine ocular surface diseases, including corneal ulceration or immune-mediated keratitis, or intraocular diseases such as uveitis. The use of blood-derived products such as serum or platelet-rich plasma, mesenchymal stem cells, or amniotic membrane grafts may be beneficial for the treatment of ulcerative and chronic keratitis in horses. Furthermore, the use of stem cells or gene therapy has promise for the treatment of Intraocular diseases such as equine recurrent uveitis by providing efficacious, practical, and long-term therapy for these blinding diseases.

Use of Biologics and Stem Cells in the Treatment of Other Inflammatory Diseases in the Horse **553**

Jennifer G. Barrett and Elizabeth S. MacDonald

Mesenchymal stem cells (MSCs) are powerful immunomodulatory cells that act via multiple mechanisms to coordinate, inhibit, and control the cells of the immune system. MSCs act as rescuers for various damaged or degenerated cells of the body via (1) cytokines, growth factors, and signaling molecules; (2) extracellular vesicle (exosome) signaling; and (3) direct donation of mitochondria. Several studies evaluating the efficacy of MSCs have used MSCs grown using xenogeneic media, which may reduce or eliminate efficacy. Although more research is needed to optimize the anti-inflammatory potential of MSCs, there is ample evidence that MSC therapeutics are worthy of further development.

Antimicrobial Properties of Equine Stromal Cells and Platelets and Future Directions **565**

Lynn M. Pezzanite, Lyndah Chow, Steven W. Dow, Laurie R. Goodrich, Jessica M. Gilbertie, and Lauren V. Schnabel

Increasing antimicrobial resistance in veterinary practice has driven the investigation of novel therapeutic strategies including regenerative and biologic therapies to treat bacterial infection. Integration of biological approaches such as platelet lysate and mesenchymal stromal cell (MSC) therapy may represent adjunctive treatment strategies for bacterial infections that minimize systemic side effects and local tissue toxicity associated with traditional antibiotics and that are not subject to antibiotic resistance. In this review, we will discuss mechanisms by which biological therapies exert antimicrobial effects, as well as potential applications and challenges in clinical implementation in equine practice.

VETERINARY CLINICS OF NORTH AMERICA: EQUINE PRACTICE

FORTHCOMING ISSUES

April 2024
Toxicologic Disorders
Megan Romano, *Editor*

August 2024
A Problem-Oriented Approach to Immunodeficiencies and Immune-Mediated Conditions in Horses
Lais R. R. Costa, *Editor*

December 2024
Equine Oncology
Anna Hollis, *Editor*

RECENT ISSUES

August 2023
Equine Colic
Louise L. Southwood, *Editor*

April 2023
Equine Infectious Diseases
Brett A. Sponseller, *Editor*

December 2022
Integrative Therapies
Kevin K. Haussler, *Editor*

SERIES OF RELATED INTEREST

Veterinary Clinics of North America: Food Animal Practice
https://www.vetfood.theclinics.com/

Preface
Considerations for the Use of Biologic and Regenerative Therapies in Equine Practice

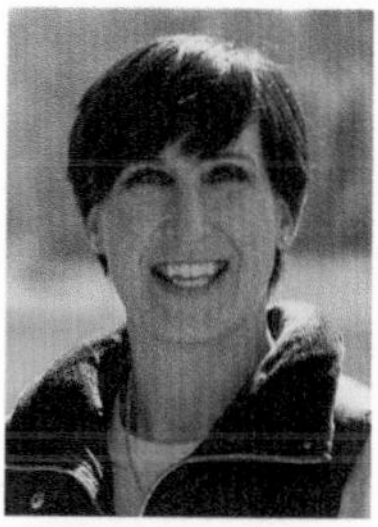

Lauren V. Schnabel, DVM, PhD, DACVS, DACVSMR
Editor

Biologic and regenerative therapies are commonly used in equine practice, yet many questions remain among practitioners regarding their use and safety. The purpose of this issue is to explain what the main biologic and regenerative therapies are in terms of their composition and mechanism of action as well as evidence to date for how they should be used, how they interact with other treatment modalities, and how to monitor response to treatment. While most of the issue focuses on musculoskeletal applications, other indications for the use of biologic and regenerative therapies are discussed, including wounds, ophthalmologic conditions, and other inflammatory diseases. Last, the antimicrobial properties of stem/stromal cells and platelets are reviewed based on mounting evidence in the recent literature.

I would like to thank Dr Tom Divers for the invitation to edit and contribute to this issue as well as Ann Gielou M. Posedio and Akshay Samson at Elsevier for their guidance and technical support. Importantly, I would also like to thank each author, recognized as an expert in the subject matter they contributed, for their time and dedication to this issue and to the advancement of equine veterinary medicine.

Vet Clin Equine 39 (2023) xiii–xiv
https://doi.org/10.1016/j.cveq.2023.07.001

I am extremely grateful for their efforts and am confident that this issue of *Veterinary Clinics of North America: Equine Practice* will serve as a valuable resource to equine practitioners and trainees for many years to come.

Lauren V. Schnabel, DVM, PhD, DACVS, DACVSMR
Department of Clinical Sciences
North Carolina State University
College of Veterinary Medicine
1060 William Moore Drive
CVM Main Building D332
Raleigh, NC 27607, USA

E-mail address:
lvschnab@ncsu.edu

Dedications

This issue is dedicated to Dr Alan Nixon, BVSc, MS, Diplomate, ACVS (1955–2023). Alan was a true horseman and a pioneer in the fields of equine musculoskeletal regenerative therapies and orthopedic surgery. He was an outstanding mentor, teacher, colleague, and friend to so many of us that worked with him at Cornell University and beyond, and will be greatly missed.

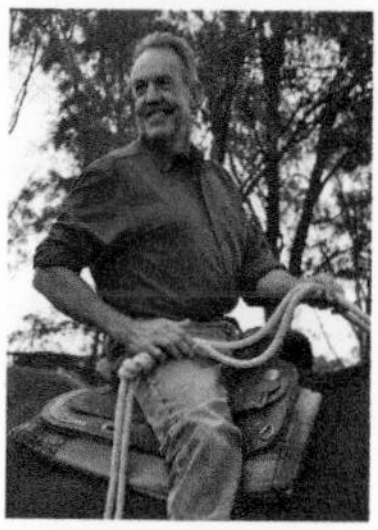

Vet Clin Equine 39 (2023) xv
https://doi.org/10.1016/j.cveq.2023.07.005
0749-0739/23/© 2023 Published by Elsevier Inc.
vetequine.theclinics.com

Introduction to Equine Biologic and Regenerative Therapies

Lindsey Boone, DVM, PhD, DACVS-LA[a,*], John Peroni, DVM, MS, DACVS[b]

KEYWORDS

- Equine • Regenerative medicine • Orthobiologics • Autologous conditioned serum
- Platelet-rich plasma • Platelet lysate • Autologous protein solution • Stem cell
- Mesenchymal stem cell

KEY POINTS

- Regenerative medicine therapeutic use is growing in equine practice and it is important that practitioners be familiar with and have a basic understanding of available products.
- Autologous conditioned serum, platelet-rich plasma, platelet lysate, and autologous protein solution are all minimally processed orthobiologics obtained from blood.
- Bone marrow aspirate, bone marrow aspirate concentrate, and adipose-derived stromal vascular fraction are obtained after tissue is harvested and processed, releasing a concentrated cell population with minimal processing.
- Culture-expanded stem cells are manipulated in culture, establishing a desired stem cell phenotype. Stem cells exert their effects at the site through paracrine signaling.

INTRODUCTION TO EQUINE BIOLOGIC AND REGENERATIVE THERAPIES

Introduction

Regenerative medicine is defined as the "process of replacing or regenerating cells, tissues, or organs to restore or establish normal function."[1] This broad field has gained significant momentum in equine veterinary medicine specifically in the treatment of damaged musculoskeletal tissues with a limited capacity for intrinsic healing such as cartilage, tendons, ligaments, and meniscus. The term "orthobiologics" has become more commonly, and more appropriately used to encompass the biologics used to assist in musculoskeletal recovery. According to the National Football League Physician Society Orthobiologics Consensus Statement, "orthobiologics" is not

[a] Department of Clinical Sciences, Auburn University College of Veterinary Medicine, John Thomas Vaughan Large Animal Teaching Hospital, 1500 Wire Road, Auburn, AL 36849, USA; [b] Department of Large Animal Medicine, University of Georgia College of Veterinary Medicine, 501 D.W. Brooks Drive, Athens, GA 30602, USA
* Corresponding author.
E-mail address: lhb0021@auburn.edu

Vet Clin Equine 39 (2023) 419–427
https://doi.org/10.1016/j.cveq.2023.06.006
0749-0739/23/Published by Elsevier Inc.

narrowly limited to a specific product but is defined as techniques and procedures designed to manufacture and deliver platelet-rich plasma (PRP) or stem cells derived from bone marrow, amnios, or adipose tissue.[2] Additionally, in equine orthopedics, the orthobiologics landscape includes other preparations such as bone marrow aspirate (BMA), bone marrow aspirate concentrate (BMAC), autologous conditioned serum (ACS), and autologous protein solution (APS). Despite this categorization, the exact formulation of each orthobiologic, the possible conditions for that they are useful, and the setting of their optimal application share *uncertainty* as an unifying commonality.[3] Considering that the effects of these products are multifactorial and not entirely understood and that the veterinary community is still lacking appropriate clinical information, orthobiologics should continue to be meticulously assessed with carefully designed clinical trials aimed at assessing their clinical value in the context of the accepted standard of care.

MINIMALLY PROCESSED BLOOD-DERIVED ORTHOBIOLOGICS

Blood-derived orthobiologics are manufactured after collecting blood from the eventual recipient of the final product. With few exceptions, these preparations are obtained with minimal processing outside of the recipient and are intended for autologous use. As a rule, blood is either collected in the presence of an anticoagulant to achieve a plasma product such as PRP and APS or is allowed to clot and then separate serum as a final product, as in the case of ACS. The collected blood is further processed to separate the liquid from the solid components of blood. This is achieved by centrifugation, gravity filtration, or a combination of both. During this processing the desired blood components of the orthobiologic are captured for therapeutic use. Equipment used for processing are meant to be simple and straight forward, requiring little to no technial expertise from the practioner, allowing these producuts to be manufactured rapidly and conveniently, stall-side. Unfortunately, there are significant differences in the equipment that is used to manipulate blood and achieve the final product. The type of equipment, the starting blood volume, any blood activation mechanism, the specifics regarding time and speed of centrifugation, and the type of filtration system used play a major role in determining the characteristics of the final product. These factors result in major challenges in our collective ability to provide a uniform and consistent assessment of the benefits and detriments of using blood-derived orthobiologics in our equine patients.

Autologous Conditioned Serum

ACS has gained widespread popularity in the management of synovial inflammation in horses. Veterinarians have become accustomed to this biological product as a treatment option for arthritis and tenosynovitis both in the management of horses with performance limitations and in the postoperative management of horses undergoing arthroscopy and tenoscopy. The premise for this treatment is that acute joint inflammation driven primarily by IL-1 and TNF-α contributes to the progressive downfall of the articular cartilage and over time joint degradation and osteoarthritis. Over the last few decades, method refinements have led to the development of specific blood collection techniques aimed at stimulating leukocytes, especially monocytes, to produce disease-modifying cytokines such as IL-1 receptor antagonist (IL-1ra) and others, including IL-10 and anabolic growth factors such as transforming growth factor-beta (TGFβ) and insulin growth factor 1 (IGF-1). Even though the exact mechanism behind this treatment modality has not been completely clarified, these anti-inflammatory cytokines benefit the synovial environment by counteracting inflammatory processes especially those driven by IL-1. Once manufactured, ACS is conveniently stored in a household freezer and maintains its cytokine profile for a long time allowing veterinarians to perform repeated treatments as needed. Even though injection protocols may be highly variable depending on the target and the veterinarian's experience, most of the time, practitioners will perform a series of injections 1 week apart for 3 to 5 treatments.

Platelet-rich Plasma

PRP has a long history in the medical field and has been applied in maxillofacial and periodontal surgery since the 1980s. Platelets, also called thrombocytes, develop from the bone marrow. Platelets are nucleated, discoid cells with different sizes and a density of approximately 2 μm in diameter, the smallest density of all blood cells. The physiological count of platelets circulating in equine blood ranges from 100,000 to 200,000 platelets per microliter. Platelets contain several secretory granules that are crucial to platelet function. There are 3 types of granules: dense granules, α-granules, and lysosomes. Platelets are primarily responsible for the aggregation process contributing to homeostasis through the processes of adhesion, activation, and aggregation. During a vascular lesion, platelets are activated, and their granules release factors that promote coagulation.[4]

Platelets were thought to have only hemostatic activity, although, in recent years, scientific research and technology have provided a new perspective on platelets and their functions. Studies suggest that platelets contain an abundance of growth factors and cytokines that can affect inflammation, angiogenesis, stem cell migration, and cell proliferation.[5] These features of PRP are somewhat captured in other terms used to define this orthobiologic such as platelet-rich growth factors, platelet-rich fibrin matrix, and platelet concentrate. This nomenclature gives us an indication of the medical rationale for its use in clinical practice. At the simplest level, the process involves collecting platelets and concentrating them to subsequently deliver the concentrate to the injured tissue thereby introducing a milieu of growth factors and proteins capable of guiding the healing response. The use of PRP in human sports medicine has attracted widespread attention in the media and has been extensively used in this field to include the treatment of tendonitis and desmitis in the equine athlete.

PRP is a natural source of signaling molecules, and on activation of platelets in PRP, the P-granules are degranulated and release growth factors and cytokines that will modify the pericellular microenvironment. Some of the most important factors released by platelets in PRP include vascular endothelial growth factor, fibroblast growth factor, platelet-derived growth factor, epidermal growth factor, hepatocyte growth factor, insulin-like growth factor 1, 2 (IGF-1, IGF-2), matrix metalloproteinases 2, 9, and interleukin 8.[6,7]

PRP plays a role in the treatment of osteoarthritis, in fact, a specific manufacturing process formed the basis for the development of APS as another autologous blood-derived product used for the treatment of osteoarthritis in horses. Similarities exist between ACS and APS because both include the concentration of IL-1ra as an important feature. Additionally, however, the APS manufacturing process includes a separator that sequesters white blood cells and platelets that are then transferred to an APS concentrator. The APS concentrator filters the product through polyacrylamide beads and desiccates it, resulting in a concentrated solution of WBCs, platelets, and plasma proteins.[8]

Despite an early publication regarding the use of APS in horses and sharp contrast with the widespread clinical use of this product, no additional follow-up clinical studies have occurred to further refine the use of APS for the treatment of equine joint disease.

Platelet Lysate

Platelet lysate (PL), otherwise known as platelet releasate, is the product of processing a platelet concentrate to obtain a final preparation that contains all the platelet injury modifying factors outlined above but that is free of cellular debris. The absence of platelets may allow the use of PL from donors in recipients of the same species and, although scientific discovery is still in its infancy, PL seems to not elicit an immune response and has been shown to exert a powerful inhibition of cell-mediated inflammatory responses.[9] Specifically, TNF-α produced by LPS-stimulated monocytes decreased over a thousand-fold in the presence of PL compared with those incubated in the presence of serum.[9] Even though PL has not been extensively studied as an orthobiologic, it is likely to contain the elements that have distinguished PRP in the treatment of soft tissue injuries and other forms of orthopedic trauma. Therefore, it would not be surprising if PL garnered a similar level of attention from veterinary professionals.

Finally, PL has recently captured the interest of the veterinary scientific community because of its reported antimicrobial effects. In addition to their well-known role as regulators of thrombosis and inflammation, there is mounting evidence to suggest that platelets play a central role in the host's response to infection.[10] Platelets kill bacteria by producing antimicrobial oxygen metabolites such as superoxide, hydrogen peroxide, and hydroxyl free radicals.[11] Moreover, platelets participate in antibody-dependent cell cytotoxicity against microbial pathogens. These effects are thought to be mediated either by a direct interaction between platelets and bacteria or, perhaps more interestingly, via peptides released by activated platelets.[12] In fact, a broad-spectrum antibacterial effect has been attributed to a select group of peptides including platelet factor 4, beta-defensin 1, and connective tissue activating peptide 3.[13,14]

TISSUE-DERIVED ORTHOBIOLOGICS: MINIMALLY MANIPULATED AND CULTURE EXPANDED

Tissue-derived orthobiologics are delivered following the collection of donor tissue. The donor tissue is processed to concentrate the cells from the collected tissue which are then either delivered to the recipient as a concentrated cellular product or the cellular population is placed in culture for expansion. The population of cells that is concentrated following tissue processing is diverse, containing several different types of cells. However, stem cells are the desired cell in this population for therapy, yet stem cells represent only a small portion of the concentrated cells that are delivered. BMAC and adipose-derived stromal vascular fraction (ADSVF) are the 2 concentrated cellular products most commonly used by equine practitioners. These products are attractive to equine practitioners because the tissues can be easily harvested, processed, and re-implanted stall-side with little-to-no delay in treatment. When the harvested cellular population obtained from the tissues is placed in culture, stem cells become established because media and growth conditions are chosen to favor stem cell growth in culture over time. The stem cells are manipulated and grown in culture to obtain the desired number of cells with the desired phenotype. This process can take several weeks following tissue harvest. When ready, the cells are harvested from the culture and then delivered to the recipient. Culture expansion allows the delivery of a greater number of stem cells than concentrated cellular products, usually 10 million stem cells or more constitute a stem cell dose. Culture expansion also allows the delivery of a more homogenous population of stem cells than concentration alone, though some diversity in cellular phenotype following culture remains.[15] Ideally the delivered cells would undergo testing (characterization) to ensure that the cells are actually stem cells before therapy, this should be the case in experimental studies, but is rarely the case in commercially grown stem cells if used in an autologous manner. The minimum criteria for characterization of MSCs include demonstration of plastic adherence, expression and lack of expression of certain surface markers, and demonstration of trilineage differentiation.[16] It is important to understand that differences in tissue source; donor age, donor health status, donor relation to the recipient, and culture methods including isolation and expansion as well as harvest and delivery techniques result in stem cells with differing therapeutic potential.[17] In addition, these stem cells are being used therapeutically to treat a variety of conditions with differing levels of severity. These factors make it challenging for practitioners to understand exactly what these therapies are doing for their patients and how they are meant to use them.

STEM CELL THERAPY: CELLULAR CONCENTRATES

Bone Marrow Aspirate and Bone Marrow Aspirate Concentrate

BMA contains a rich milieu of platelets, red blood cells, white blood cells, hematopoietic and non-hematopoietic precursor cells that include stem cells, as well as several important anabolic growth factors, cytokines, and chemokines important for tissue repair. The aspirate can be further concentrated via centrifugation using either density gradient media or a gravitational separation device. Concentration of BMA yields a product with a higher number of nucleated cells including progenitor and stem cells, growth factors, cytokines, and platelets.[18] This product is referred to as BMAC. It is important to recognize that although concentration results in a greater percentage of mesenchymal stem cells (MSCs), the number of cells within BMAC remains low, approximately 0.001% to 0.01% of the mononuclear cell population of BMAC are MSCs.[18] Despite the low MSC population, BMAC has been shown to have reparative, anabolic effects experimentally on musculoskeletal tissues.[18,19] Most equine research has centered on the use of BMAC for the treatment of suspensory ligament desmopathy while clinically, treatment of naturally occurring acute and chronic suspensory desmopathy with BMAC has proved promising.[20,21]

Adipose-derived Stromal Vascular Fraction

ADSVF is a cellular product obtained from adipose tissue. Adipose is harvested stall-side from the patient via either lipoaspiration or lipectomy. The adipose aspirate or tissue is then subjected to enzymatic digestion or mechanical agitation followed by centrifugation resulting in an aqueous fluid with a concentrated cellular pellet, termed the stromal vascular fraction.[22] The cellular pellet contains a heterogenous population of cells that includes endothelial cells, monocytes, lymphocytes, myeloid cells, pericytes, and hematopoietic stem cells.[22] Adipose tissue has a greater number of MSCs within tissue, therefore the MSC yield is greater than BMAC.[23] Currently, this product requires shipment of the adipose tissue to an approved commercial laboratory for processing. Cells are typically shipped back within 48 hours for treatment. There are currently no commercially available medical devices to produce ADSVF stall-side for the equine patient which differs from BMAC.

STEM CELL THERAPY: CULTURE EXPANSION

Stem cells are immature, unspecialized cells with the capacity for self-renewal and differentiation. Differentiation is the process by which the cell changes to a more mature, specialized cell. Stem cells are found in limited quantities in all body tissues and are responsible for replacing injured, diseased, or aged stromal cells.

Stem cell therapy was first introduced because of the stem cells self-renewal and differentiation capacity. MSCs were injected into the site of injury and thought to integrate and differentiate into the desired tissue. However, studies have shown that MSC engraftment, retention, and direct differentiation are limited.[15] Despite this, improvement in clinical signs of the patient and quality of repair tissue have been reported. Therefore, our current understanding is that the injected MSCs interact with native cells within the injured environment via cell–cell interactions and secreted factors (paracrine signaling). These interactions modulate the wound environment to a more immunotolerant that aids rather than hinders tissue repair by native cells.[15]

Stem cells are categorized based on various criteria including their differentiation capacity (potency), tissue of origin, and relationship to the recipient of cellular therapy (autologous, allogenic, and xenogeneic). Stem cells can be obtained from various stages of organismal development that determines their potency. Cells can be totipotent, pluripotent, multipotent, oligopotent, bipotent, or unipotent.[24] Totipotent cells can form any tissue in the body and are derived from the fertilized ovum whereas pluripotent cells are obtained from the embryo and can emerge into cells of all 3 germ layers.[24] Pluripotent stem cells can be obtained either from the embryo termed embryonic stem cells (ESCs) or cells can be obtained from somatic tissues and re-programed to an embryonic state, termed induced pluripotent stem cells (iPSCs). Multipotent cells only differentiate into cells of the germ layer from which the cell was obtained. These are the most common type of cells used for therapy in veterinary medicine.[24] Multipotent stem cells are commonly obtained from connective (mesenchymal) tissue and can differentiate into another type of connective tissue and are termed MSCs.[24] Differentiation of MSCs into the 3 tissues: bone, fat, and cartilage is termed trilineage differentiation and this is one of the criteria used to characterize cultured cells as MSCs. Oligopotent, bipotent, and unipotent cells are obtained from the target tissue and can only produce cells of the specific tissue from which they were obtained. As the cells lose potency, they also lose the capacity for self-renewal, meaning that totipotent or pluripotent stem cells have a greater capacity for replication than multipotent stem cells. Although ESC and iPSCs have been successfully obtained and cultured from horses, MSCs from fetal or adult tissue remain the most common type of stem cell therapy used in equine practice.[25]

MSCs can be obtained from either fetal or adult tissues. Fetal tissues used in practice may include placental tissue, umbilical cord blood, or umbilical cord tissue. These tissues are obtained from the fetus at the time of birth, processed, and then banked for future use. More commonly, MSCs are obtained from adult tissues such as peripheral blood MSCs, adipose SCs, or bone marrow (BMSCs). In equine practice, adipose tissue and bone marrow are the most commonly harvested tissues for concentration or culture expansion of MSCs.[25,26] Bone marrow is harvested either from the sternum or the tuber coxae based on clinician preference and comfort. Adipose is harvested via an open technique or through a small stab incision with insertion and redirection of a lipoaspiration needle just lateral to the tailhead. Of these 2 tissues, BMSCs are the most commonly researched MSC in veterinary medicine[24] and the most commonly used MSC therapy in equine practice.[26]

Another consideration for MSC therapy is the tissue donor. Tissue can be obtained from the patient (autologous), a donor different from the patient but of the same species (allogenic), or a donor from a different species (xenogenic). Autologous tissue is commonly used in equine practice, however, when growing cells in culture there can be significant delays in treatment (~4 weeks) when using autologous cells. In addition, the age and disease status of the patient can change the self-renewal and differentiation capacity of the cells. Allogenic cells are an attractive alternative because cells can be harvested from young, healthy donors, expanded in culture, and characterized for phenotype and function. These culture expanded characterized cells are stored for rapid use with little-to-no delay of treatment. Allogenic use in the horse has been investigated because MSCs are considered hypoimmunogenic due to their low expression of major histocompatibility complex II.[15] Despite this, both cellular and humoral immune responses to administered allogeneic stem cells have been observed.[15]

As previously stated, of the factors secreted from MSCs play a major role in tissue repair. These secreted factors, termed the secretome, are gaining interest as an additional avenue of stem cell therapy. The secretome consists of cytokines, chemokines, growth factors, extracellular vesicles, lectins, prostaglandins, and enzymes from MSCs.[17] Extracellular vesicles are membrane-bound vesicles important in cellular signaling that contain several bioactive factors including mRNAs, microRNAs, cytokines, and other proteins.[17] MSCs can be manipulated in culture via serum starvation, hypoxia, and induced inflammation (priming) to produce different secreted factors in the culture media that can be harvested and used for therapy.[27]

SUMMARY

The use of regenerative medicine in equine practice is increasing. Yet there is no clear understanding of each product's specific mechanism of action, treatment efficacy, or best treatment practices. To address some of these challenges, standards defining each therapeutic and its components continue to be refined. These standards need to be measured and reported within the scientific literature to understand the similarities and differences of each therapy. Finally, to understand treatment efficacy, more well-designed, properly powered, placebo-controlled studies are needed. Regenerative medicine holds great promise for our equine patients.

DISCLOSURE

The Authors have nothing to disclose.

REFERENCES

1. Daar AS, Greenwood HL. A proposed definition of regenerative medicine. Journal of Tissue Engineering and Regenerative Medicine 2007;1:179–84.
2. Rodeo SA, Bedi A. 2019-2020 NFL and NFL physician society orthobiologics consensus statement. Sports Health 2020;12:58–60.
3. Sampson S, Vincent H, Ambach M. Education and standardization of orthobiologics: Past, present & future. Platelet Rich Plasma in Orthopaedics and Sports Medicine 2018;277–87.
4. Theml H. Physiology and pathophysiology of blood cells. New York: Color Atlas of Hematology Stuttgart, Thieme; 2004.
5. Harmon K, Hanson R, Bowen J, et al. Guidelines for the use of platelet rich plasma. Available at: https://www.scribd.com/document/159334949/206-ICMS-Guidelines-for-the-Use-of-Platelet-Rich-Plasma-Draftob-oasbonasdandbowndoww. 2011.
6. Andia I, Abate M. Platelet-rich plasma: underlying biology and clinical correlates. Regenerative medicine 2013;8:645–58.

7. Andrae J, Gallini R, Betsholtz C. Role of platelet-derived growth factors in physiology and medicine. Genes Dev 2008;22:1276–312.
8. Bertone AL, Ishihara A, Zekas LJ, et al. Evaluation of a single intra-articular injection of autologous protein solution for treatment of osteoarthritis in horses. Am J Vet Res 2014;75:141–51.
9. Naskou MC, Norton NA, Copland IB, et al. Innate immune responses of equine monocytes cultured in equine platelet lysate. Vet Immunol Immunopathol 2018;195:65–71.
10. Jenne CN, Kubes P. Platelets in inflammation and infection. Platelets 2015;26:286–92.
11. Ali RA, Wuescher LM, Dona KR, et al. Platelets mediate host defense against Staphylococcus aureus through direct bactericidal activity and by enhancing macrophage activities. J Immunol 2017;198:344–51.
12. Cox D. Bacteria-platelet interactions. J Thromb Haemostasis 2009;7:1865.
13. Palankar R, Kohler T, Krauel K, et al. Platelets kill bacteria by bridging innate and adaptive immunity via platelet factor 4 and FcγRIIA. J Thromb Haemostasis 2018;16:1187–97.
14. Kraemer BF, Campbell RA, Schwertz H, et al. Novel anti-bacterial activities of β-defensin 1 in human platelets: suppression of pathogen growth and signaling of neutrophil extracellular trap formation. PLoS Pathog 2011;7:e1002355.
15. Fortier LA, Goodrich LR, Ribitsch I, et al. One health in regenerative medicine: report on the second Havemeyer symposium on regenerative medicine in horses. Regen Med 2020;15:1775–87.
16. Dominici M, Le Blanc K, Mueller I, et al. Minimal criteria for defining multipotent mesenchymal stromal cells. The International Society for Cellular Therapy position statement. Cytotherapy 2006;8:315–7.
17. Williams KB, Ehrhart NP. Regenerative medicine 2.0: extracellular vesicle–based therapeutics for musculoskeletal tissue regeneration. J Am Vet Med Assoc 2022;260:683–9.
18. Fortier LA, Potter HG, Rickey EJ, et al. Concentrated bone marrow aspirate improves full-thickness cartilage repair compared with microfracture in the equine model. JBJS 2010;92:1927–37.
19. Ross MW, Smith RKW, Smith JJ. Anabolic effects of acellular bone marrow, platelet rich plasma, and serum on equine suspensory ligament fibroblasts in vitro. Vet Comp Orthop Traumatol 2006;19:43–7.
20. Herthel DJ. Enhanced suspensory ligament healing in 100 horses by stem cells and other bone marrow components. AAEP proceedings 2001;47:319–21.
21. Maleas G, Mageed M. Effectiveness of platelet-rich plasma and bone marrow aspirate concentrate as treatments for chronic hindlimb proximal suspensory desmopathy. Front Vet Sci 2021;8:678453.
22. Bora P, Majumdar AS. Adipose tissue-derived stromal vascular fraction in regenerative medicine: a brief review on biology and translation. Stem Cell Res Ther 2017;8:1–10.
23. Metcalf GL, McClure SR, Hostetter JM, et al. Evaluation of adipose-derived stromal vascular fraction from the lateral tailhead, inguinal region, and mesentery of horses. Can J Vet Res 2016;80:294–301.
24. El-Husseiny HM, Mady EA, Helal MAY, et al. The pivotal role of stem cells in veterinary regenerative medicine and tissue engineering. Veterinary Sciences 2022;9:648.

25. Velloso Alvarez A, Boone LH, Braim AP, et al. A survey of clinical usage of non-steroidal intra-articular therapeutics by equine practitioners. Front Vet Sci 2020;7:579967.
26. Knott LE, Fonseca-Martinez BA, O'Connor AM, et al. Current use of biologic therapies for musculoskeletal disease: a survey of board-certified equine specialists. Vet Surg 2022;51:557–67.
27. Harman RM, Churchill KA, Jager MC, et al. The equine mesenchymal stromal cell secretome inhibits equid herpesvirus type 1 strain Ab4 in epithelial cells. Res Vet Sci 2021;141:76–80.

Equine Platelet-Rich Plasma

Taralyn M. McCarrel, DVM, DACVS-LA

KEYWORDS

- Platelet-rich plasma • Tendon • Ligament • Cartilage • Joint • Biologic
- Regenerative • Growth factor

KEY POINTS

- Platelet-rich plasma (PRP) is a safe but highly variable orthobiologic which has made drawing firm conclusions on the optimal preparation and treatment protocol from the literature difficult.
- Pooled allogeneic cell-free platelet lysates or freeze-dried PRP likely represent the future of PRP therapy due to increased convenience, and product characteristics that can be more clearly defined and controlled before treatment.
- PRP continues to hold promise for treatment of tendon and ligament injuries, for osteoarthritis management which should perhaps be focused on long-term outcomes in early disease, and the exciting potential as an adjunct to treatment of septic arthritis.

INTRODUCTION

Platelet-rich plasma (PRP) has been used principally as an orthobiologic therapy in equine practice for approximately 20 years. Among the orthobiologic therapies currently in use, it is one of the most largely studied in the basic science, veterinary, and human medical literature. A PubMed search using the search terms "platelet rich plasma AND (regen* OR biologic* OR orthobiologic* OR growth factor*)" yields 6020 publications to date which dwarfs similar literature searches for all other orthobiologic therapies combined with the exception of mesenchymal stem cells. In spite of these efforts, numerous questions and controversies remain. The abundant sources or variability in outcomes based on the donor, preparation method, activation state, treatment method and schedule, disease or injury state, and outcome assessment methodology can feel insurmountable at times.[1] This high variability in addition to continued incomplete reporting in the scientific literature despite publications calling for standardization in reporting[1,2] has stymied progress in the understanding of the optimal composition and therapeutic approach to maximize efficacy. The rationale for use of PRP and discussion of PRP definitions will be reviewed. Then, the clinical use of PRP based on recent surveys of equine veterinarians will be discussed in light

Department of Large Animal Clinical Sciences, University of Florida College of Veterinary Medicine, 2015 Southwest 16th Avenue, Gainesville, FL 32608, USA
E-mail address: tmccarrel@ufl.edu

Vet Clin Equine 39 (2023) 429–442
https://doi.org/10.1016/j.cveq.2023.06.007

of the available literature. Finally, the anticipated future evolution of PRP and new therapeutic uses will be introduced.

RATIONALE AND DEFINITIONS

The most basic definition of PRP is a plasma preparation that has an increased platelet concentration compared with whole blood. The theoretic basis for the use of PRP to improve repair of musculoskeletal tissues was initially focused on the growth factors contained within platelet-alpha granules which have been shown to exert a wide range of reparative effects.[3,4] However, the bioactive factors in PRP are far more complex than the lists of growth factors provided in many publications. Rather, the sum and relative proportions of the total bioactive molecules of the product must be considered. These factors are derived from the platelets, white blood cells (WBC), red blood cells, and plasma proteins within PRP. This combination of factors includes pro-inflammatory and anti-inflammatory cytokines, anabolic growth factors and catabolic enzymes, hormones, acute phase proteins, and immunoglobulins, among others.[5] The concentration of some of the constituents of PRP has been shown to produce different effects on cells and tissues and led to the development of several classification systems.[6–11]

Dohan Ehrenfest and colleagues classified PRP into four groups based on leukocyte concentration and activation state.[12] The four categories are (1) pure PRP which has low WBC and is not activated, (2) leukocyte-rich PRP which has high WBC and is not activated, (3) pure platelet-rich fibrin which has low WBC and is activated, and (4) leukocyte-rich platelet-rich fibrin which has high WBC and is activated. Numerous synonyms are used in the literature such as leukocyte-reduced or leukocyte-poor PRP which are analogous to pure PRP as an example. Since the four-part classification scheme was developed, several new schemes have been reported totaling nine different classifications methods.[13] The number of different classification schemes is due in part to the evolution of slightly different methods to produce PRP, recognition of the importance of different factors, as well as development of platelet concentrates that share properties of PRP and are often incorrectly identified as a PRP product. There are 50 different PRP preparation systems available as well as a multitude of manual preparation protocols reported.[13] Hessel and colleagues compared three different PRP preparation systems and one manual PRP preparation method in horses.[14] The study also evaluated a filtration-based platelet and WBC concentrate that is free of plasma and therefore should not be considered PRP as plasma proteins are an important component of PRP. Equine platelets concentrated to a lesser degree than what was reported for human blood for all systems investigated. This emphasizes an important point that each methodology and system must be validated for each species of interest. In addition, only two systems significantly increased platelet concentration above baseline blood concentrations, and for two systems at least one of six horses actually had lower platelet concentration in the final product indicating PRP had not been produced.[14] This further emphasizes the critical need for all research studies to report the characterization of every PRP sample used in the study as some preparations will inevitably fail and treatment with failed product should be excluded from results.

PRP may be frozen and thawed either for the purpose of storage of additional aliquots from a single prep, for the purpose of cell and platelet lysis and therefore protein release, for mass production of allogeneic off-the-shelf products to be used directly as therapeutics, or for xenogen-free stem cell isolation and expansion. These preparations should be referred to as platelet lysates (PLs), leaving PRP to refer to treatment with fresh product. A single immediate freeze–thaw cycle to release intracellular proteins did not reduce the concentrations of any protein measured relative to fresh, bovine thrombin-activated equine PRP.[15] When PRP was stored frozen in a −20°C automatic defrost freezer, −20°C manual defrost freezer, −80°C manual defrost freezer, or liquid nitrogen, insulin-like growth factor (IGF-1) was reduced compared with baseline in all conditions. Platelet-derived growth factor and transforming growth factor remained at baseline concentrations for 1 month at −80°C and 6 months in liquid nitrogen.[15] Lyophilization, also known as freeze drying, may have an added benefit of prolonged shelf-life at room temperature which is more practical in a field service setting. Even among PLs and lyophilized PLs, there is much variation in production methods with various preparations including or excluding WBC, plasma proteins, and or fragments of lysed cells and platelets. The desire to retain or eliminate plasma proteins is an important area for consideration. Numerous PRP focused publications list IGF-1 among the growth factors concentrated in platelet α-granules; however, this is incorrect. IGF-1 is a hormone produced by the liver and is predominantly present in the plasma portion of PRP.[5] The increased concentration of platelets in PRP does not result in increased IGF-1 concentrations compared with platelet-poor plasma.[16] Thus, plasma-free PL will be depleted of IGF-1. A study focused on developing PL for antimicrobial activity found that maintaining plasma proteins in the preparation was critical for optimal antimicrobial function,[17] whereas another focused on developing an equine PL as a cross-species therapeutic and emphasized removal of cellular fragments and plasma proteins to limit the risk of immune response to the therapy.[18] PLs or lyophilized PL have many potential advantages over PRP, which will be addressed further in the future directions section.

CLINICAL USE OF PLATELET-RICH PLASMA

The proportion of equine practitioners using orthobiologics in their practice that include PRP in their therapeutic armamentarium is reported to be 77.3% in one survey of equine practitioners (general and specialist) predominantly practicing in the United States[19] and 87.5% of diplomates of the American College of Veterinary Surgeons or American College of Sports Medicine and Rehabilitation.[20] The most common indication for PRP therapy and mode of delivery were tendon and ligament lesions (67% of respondents) and intralesional injection (97% of respondents), respectively.[19,20] For equine practitioners, the median rank choice for intra-articular therapies ranked corticosteroids first, hyaluronic acid second, and autologous conditioned serum, autologous protein solution, and PRP all had a median rank of 4±2.[19] Among equine specialists, 68% reported using PRP for intra-articular injection.[20]

Tendon and Ligament Lesions

The in vitro, in vivo, and clinical investigation of PRP in horses was initially focused on ligamentous and tendinous lesions; thus, the more frequent use by equine practitioners for these indications is expected. Allogeneic frozen-thawed PRP was applied to superficial digital flexor tendon (SDFT)[16] and suspensory ligament[21] explants in vitro and resulted in improved expression of anabolic genes without concurrent increase in catabolic genes, although allogeneic acellular bone marrow was superior to PRP for suspensory ligaments. A follow-up study applied fresh autologous PRP, fresh autologous bone marrow aspirate (BMA), or allogeneic lyophilized platelets to SDFT and suspensory ligament explants and found that lyophilized platelets and PRP produced improved gene expression profiles in both tissue types compared with BMA, which significantly increased catabolic enzyme expression.[22] The PRP used for the initial and follow-up studies had moderately increased platelet concentration and a WBC concentration that did not differ from baseline blood values.[16,22] The lyophilized platelets contained no WBC and the BMA were highly concentrated for nucleated cells in the fresh PRP study, and WBC were found to be correlated with increased catabolic enzyme expression.[22] The lack of live cells in the initial studies by Schnabel and colleagues[16,21] most likely explains the difference in results compared with the studies using fresh PRP,[22] which was performed to reflect the most common clinical use at the time.

In a series of publications, Bosch and colleagues described treatment of surgically created core lesions in the SDFT with PRP or placebo control in horses.[23–25] Intralesional injection of fresh, high-platelet, high WBC PRP without exogenous platelet activation resulted in increased amounts of collagen and proteoglycan, improved collagen organization on ultrasound and histology, increased vascularity on Doppler ultrasound and immunohistochemistry, and higher strength at failure and higher elastic modulus compared with control.[23–25] The increased strength at failure and elastic modulus indicates that the tendon is stiffer and could be misinterpreted as undesirable rigid scar tissue. However, when compared with previously published values for normal tendons, both PRP and placebo-treated tendons had strength at failure and elastic modulus below that of normal tendons, with PRP-treated tendons more closely approximating normal values.[26]

Although the results of in vitro and in vivo investigation in horses have been consistently positive, the results of clinical reports are less consistent (**Table 1**).[27–32] Unfortunately, clinical studies are often uncontrolled, do not report the characterization of the PRP produced and used in each case, and have variable rehabilitation within and between studies. The loss of cases due to deviations from study protocol also occurred with varying frequency among studies. All of these factors impair our ability to compare studies and draw conclusions based on the results.

Intra-articular Pathologies

The use of PRP for management of joint disease and particularly clinical studies of intra-articular use in horses has lagged far behind medical practice in people. Although significant challenges remain and results are conflicting, numerous clinical trials investigating PRP for the treatment of osteoarthritis in people have been performed. A recent review summarized the conclusions drawn based on results of these studies to be that (1) PRP is more effective in younger patients with less severe osteoarthritis, (2) although some studies show no difference in outcomes between leukocyte-rich and leukocyte-poor PRP, some studies have shown improved clinical outcomes and reduced post-injection pain when leukocyte-reduced PRP is used, (3) the onset of clinical effect of PRP is delayed compared with hyaluronic acid but PRP seems to have a longer duration of benefit.[33] We should consider these conclusions when designing clinical investigation in horses. The current equine literature is limited to small clinical reports or in vivo studies, for which a high leukocyte filtration system devoid of plasma has been used, and outcome measures are often limited to short-term evaluation (hours to days post-injection).[34–36]

PL has been shown to maintain chondrocyte phenotype in culture with increased collagen II and aggrecan expression, whereas collagen I expression was decreased compared with fetal bovine serum.[37] PL was also found to decrease concentrations of catabolic enzymes while increasing the concentration of the endogenous inhibitor of the same catabolic enzymes and increasing glycosaminoglycan concentrations in synovial fluid from osteoarthritic joints.[38] Equine PL was investigated in vitro in a model of inflamed synoviocytes. The conditioned media produced by synoviocytes with PL or platelet-poor plasma treatments were then applied to chondrocytes in vitro.[39] PL resulted in increased synoviocyte proliferation, increased hyaluronic acid production,

Table 1
Clinical studies of platelet-rich plasma for treatment of tendon and ligament injuries

Lesion	N	Randomized	Blinded	Control	PRP	Activation	Dose	Outcome	Citation
Various	99 Various	No	No	No	Manual Frozen WBC not reported	Various	Based on lesion size Intralesional and perilesional	81% return to prior work within 6 mo	Scala M et al,[27] 2014
SDFT	118 National Hunt horses	No	No	Normal racehorses Rehab only = 24 Bar firing = 38 Tendon split = 18 Tendon split + bar fire = 12 PRP = 26	Orthokine System Not characterized	Calcium chloride	Based on lesion size Intralesional	All injured has performance parameters less than normal horses No difference between treatment modality for outcome	Witte S et al,[28] 2016
Midbody suspensory ligament	9 Standardbred racehorses	No	No	Normal racehorses	Buffy coat WBC not reported	Bovine thrombin	Based on lesion size Intralesional	All returned to racing Only difference from controls was number of starts in third year and decreased earnings/start in first year	Waselau M et al,[29] 2018
Sesamoiditis	39 Thoroughbred yearlings	Yes	Yes	Saline	GPS II System high platelet high WBC system Values for study horses not reported	No	3 mL Perilesional	PRP treated more likely to start a race as 2 year old, no difference for any other parameter	Garrett KS et al,[30] 2013

(*continued on next page*)

Table 1
(continued)

Lesion	*N*	Randomized	Blinded	Control	PRP	Activation	Dose	Outcome	Citation
Proximal suspensory	100 Western performance	Yes	Yes	Extracorporeal shockwave (ESW) therapy	Arthrex autologous conditioned plasma (ACP) Low-platelet, low WBC system Not characterized in study	No	3-6 mL Intralesional or perilesional	4 d ESW decreased lameness 6-mo agent reported lameness and return to work did not differ by treatment 12-mo agent reported optimal treatment correlated with ultrasound score	Giunta K et al,[31] 2019
Chronic proximal suspensory	93 English sport horses	No	No	Rehab only = 22 Bone marrow aspirate concentrate (BMAC) = 25 E-PET system = 46	E-PET system plasma free platelet and WBC concentrate Not characterized in study	No	2-4 mL Intralesional	At 6, 12, and 18 mo percent of horses sound and in work greater for treatments vs control, for long-term BMAC had greater percentages than PRP	Maleas G et al,[32] 2021

and increased interleukin-6 production. Application of the synoviocyte conditioned media to chondrocytes resulted in increased collagen II and aggrecan gene expression, whereas matrix metalloproteinase-13 expression was decreased. These results support an anti-inflammatory, anti-catabolic, reparative effect of PL for joint disease.

Garbin and colleagues compared injection of autologous leukocyte-reduced PRP to allogeneic leukocyte-reduced freeze-dried PL in healthy equine joints.[40] Both treatments elicited a mild inflammatory response characterized by increased nucleated cell count, prostaglandin E_2, and total protein that was short-lived and self-limiting. In addition, a saline or sham injection group was not included in the study to compare the effect of arthrocentesis on these parameters. There was no difference between the two platelet products for any of the parameters evaluated indicating allogeneic freeze-dried PL may be a viable option of intra-articular injection.

Davis and colleagues investigated a variety of orthobiologics including PRP for post-operative outcome in English sport horses undergoing arthroscopic surgery for meniscal tear.[41] There was no effect of treatment with any orthobiologic on outcome. However, given the number of different treatments investigated, the treatment groups were small which may have limited power and concurrent disease factors such as radiographic changes consistent with osteoarthritis, subchondral bone cyst, and cartilage injury were not controlled for between groups. The PRP system used was reported, but the preparations used in the study were not characterized. Further controlled studies with well-characterized products and consideration of the findings in the human literature are needed before any conclusions can be drawn on the efficacy of PRP or PL for joint injection.

PLATELET ACTIVATION

The vast majority of equine practitioners (89%) reported that they do not activate PRP, 8% activate with calcium chloride, and equal proportions (4% each) reported using shock wave or freeze–thaw.[19] Bovine thrombin is among the strongest activators of equine platelets, exceeding autologous equine thrombin for growth factor release.[42] However, concerns regarding immune response to xenogenic proteins and evidence of increased inflammation when injected in joints[34] have likely limited its use in more recent years. The clotting effect stimulated by bovine thrombin is also rapid requiring the use of special dual injection syringe systems which may further limit use. The rationale for injection of resting PRP is based on the concept that exposure to collagen in injured tissues will stimulate platelet degranulation as occurs during the normal coagulation response when a wound is created. In vitro studies have supported this concept[6,22]; however, the technical challenges of measuring growth factor release in vivo have limited investigation in this area.

Physical methods of platelet activation include lysis via freeze–thaw and application of shockwave. Freeze–thaw significantly and dramatically increases growth factor release from platelets; however, shockwave was effective at increasing growth factor release above baseline values.[43] Two freeze–thaw cycles were found to result in significantly greater growth factor release than one freeze–thaw cycle; however, there was no benefit of additional freeze-thaw cycles.[44] PLs are generated following freeze–thaw and as it is anticipated that these products may become more widespread, the debate surrounding activation may become irrelevant.

CONCURRENT NONSTEROIDAL ANTI-INFLAMMATORY THERAPY

The administration of nonsteroidal anti-inflammatory drugs (NSAIDs) either before or after treatment with PRP is one of the most significant controversies surrounding this therapeutic and in contrast to the size of the debate, the least well studied. Equine practitioners reported using NSAIDs concurrently with PRP at a relatively high rate (54% of respondents) compared with what would be expected in human medicine.[19] Although the reasons for concurrent NSAID use were not reported, possible explanations may include the limited use of other forms of analgesia routinely in equine practice, that a high percentage of horses are already on NSAIDs for musculoskeletal injury, or the desire to prevent complaints about post-injection swelling or lameness from owners. The dogma that NSAIDs must not be given before or following treatment originates from human medical practice and is based on the concept that NSAIDs inhibit platelet function and thus will inhibit growth factor release. Platelets have cyclooxygenase-1 (COX-1) enzymes on the outer platelet membrane which converts arachidonic acid to thromboxane, a potent platelet activator.[45,46] Nonsteroidal anti-inflammatories, particularly those that are not COX-2 selective, reversibly bind COX-1 and reduce the production of thromboxane.[45] Although this argument based on fundamental physiology is sound, it neglects to acknowledge that platelet activation and resultant coagulation are functions critical for life and thus there are several pathways for platelet activation, some of which are not dependent on thromboxane. In addition, horses are less thromboxane-dependent than many other species for platelet activation, so what may hold true in people on this matter may not apply to the horse.[47]

Schippinger and colleagues investigated aggregation of platelets in PRP prepared from people receiving a variety of NSAID therapies.[48] When platelets were treated with arachidonic acid, aggregation was not observed and it was concluded that NSAIDs impaired the function of platelets in PRP and must be withheld before collection of blood for preparation of PRP. However, within the same study, platelets were also stimulated with collagen, adenine diphosphate (ADP), and thrombin receptor activator peptide-6 and aggregation did not differ between PRP from patients treated with NSAIDs and PRP prepared from individuals not receiving NSAIDs for any of the other activators indicating that other pathways of platelet activation remained functional in NSAID-treated PRP. Ludwig and colleagues found that treatment of dogs with a COX-2 selective NSAID had no effect on platelet degranulation in response to bovine thrombin activation, growth factor release, or systemic thromboxane concentrations as would be expected given that thrombin does not require thromboxane to stimulate platelet activation and a COX-2 selective NSAID should have minimal effect on COX-1 on platelet membranes.[49] The effect of NSAIDs on platelet function has also been investigated in horses treated with the nonselective NSAIDs phenylbutazone and flunixin meglumine, and the COX-2 selective NSAID firocoxib.[50] Firocoxib had no effect on systemic thromboxane concentrations, whereas both phenylbutazone and flunixin meglumine significantly reduced systemic thromboxane confirming COX-1 inhibition. Primary hemostasis was delayed significantly when collagen-ADP was used for activation. However, growth factor concentrations were not different compared with no treatment control following thrombin activation of platelets. Although questions remain as to whether NSAIDs may impair growth factor release in response to weak activators, strong activators and logically physical methods of platelet lysis for growth factor release are most likely unaffected.

Another critical question in the debate surrounding NSAID use that has yet to be addressed is whether administration of NSAIDs after treatment with PRP will negatively impact PRP effects. The concept that NSAIDs should be withheld is based on the concept that PRP and platelet degranulation stimulate inflammation as is the normal first step following injury and coagulation. However, several studies promote the anti-inflammatory effects of PRP. Thus, the question to be answered is, will

NSAIDs impair PRPs effects, have no impact, or work synergistically with PRPs anti-inflammatory mediators?

COMPLICATIONS

Reports of serious complications following injection of PRP are rare in veterinary and human medical literature. Equine practitioners reported experiencing no joint flares (44.9%) or less than 2% of cases with joint flares (38.8%) following PRP injection with the remainder reporting estimates of 5% (9.2%) or 10% (5.6%) of horses experiencing joint flares after PRP injection.[19] Local inflammation at the injection site was observed by 86% of equine specialists, 4.4% reported observing infection at the injection site, and less than 1% reported observing systemic inflammation following administration of PRP therapy.[20] However, the percentage of horses experiencing these complications was not reported. A clinical study investigating PRP injection for proximal suspensory ligament desmitis reported 2/10 horses experiencing heat, swelling, and increased lameness following injection that resolved with NSAID therapy.[31] The investigators postulated that the anticoagulant may have contributed to these signs and did not use anticoagulant for PRP preparation for the remainder of the study and reported no further events. It must be emphasized that the properties of the system used in this study allow PRP preparation without acid-citrate-dextrose anticoagulant, however, that is not the case for the majority of preparation methods.

FUTURE DIRECTIONS

Platelet Lysate and Freeze-Dried Platelet-Rich Plasma

The advantages that led to the rapid adoption of PRP therapy compared with some other orthobiologics are that autologous PRP can be quickly and easily prepared stall side for immediate use, whereas many other therapies require transport and incubation before injection at a later date. However, the drawbacks include donor variability, system variability, and the inability to quickly validate the quality of the PRP stall side. In addition, many systems require customized centrifuges and specialized kits to prepare PRP. These centrifuges can be cumbersome for field practitioners, and with the increasing regulatory oversight by the Food and Drug Administration, some companies with well-validated systems for horses in the literature are nevertheless refusing to continue to sell kits to veterinarians leaving the unsuspecting veterinarian with an expensive and otherwise useless piece of equipment.

In light of the drawbacks of autologous fresh PRP preparation, PL and freeze-dried PRP pose several advantages. Freeze-dried PRP and PL can be prepared from a group of disease-free donor horses to produce an off-the-shelf product that has already been tested to meet certain predefined consistency and quality standards. PLs produced from pooled PRP from several horses have been shown to have improved protein consistency and thus activity of the product.[17] The process of producing most PL results in removal of cell fragments and WBC leaving an acellular protein suspension with decreased likelihood of immune response.[18,22,39] Freeze-drying platelets or freeze-drying PL have the added advantage of increased stability, the ability to be stored at room temperature, and can be rehydrated to whatever volume and dose is desired.[18,22] A careful development of these products could aid in eliminating some of the variability that plagues our ability to make clear evidence-based decisions surrounding PRP therapy.

In the first in vitro investigation of trehalose freeze-dried platelets, growth factors were released immediately on rehydration and were highly consistent within the batch used for the study.[22] Even with rapid release and elimination of growth factors in culture with tendon and ligament explants for 4 days, gene expression patterns were favorable for tendon and ligament repair with improved collagen I to collagen III ratio and decreased matrix metalloproteinase-13 expression. A freeze-dried preparation of washed and lysed platelets following elimination of WBC was shown to suppress proliferation of activated T cells and stimulated murine peritoneal macrophages to express an M2 (anti-inflammatory) phenotype.[18] Finally, platelet proteins released in PLs have been shown to have antimicrobial properties.[51,52] Although the initial studies on the antimicrobial properties of PRP were performed decades ago, recent research is promising exciting possibilities for the treatment of septic arthritis.

Antimicrobial Effects of Platelet-Rich Plasma and Septic Arthritis

Yeaman and colleagues first demonstrated dose-dependent microbiostatic and microbiocidal activity of rabbit platelet proteins against *Staphylococcus aureus, Escherichia coli, Bacillus subtilis*, and *Candida albicans*.[52] A handful of studies investigating in vitro microbiocidal effects of human platelet proteins, PRP, and plasma proteins against isolates from infections in people and clinical reports of infected wound healing followed. The first report of the antimicrobial effects of equine PRP showed that thrombin-activated platelets had greater inhibitory effect on *E coli* than platelets that had not been activated.[53] Finally, in an elegant series of experiments, Gilbertie and colleagues took a step-wise approach to prepare a PL optimized for its antimicrobial effects.[17] The final optimized product is a pooled PRP lysate with high platelet concentration and removal of cellular elements and WBC, retention of plasma at 10% concentration, and elimination of anionic and large (>10 kDa) cationic proteins. The resultant product exhibits antibiofilm and antimicrobial activity and performs synergistically with amikacin against *S aureus, Streptococcus equi ssp zooepidemicus, E coli*, and *Pseudomonas aeruginosa*. A follow-up in vivo study compared treatment of horses with tarsocrural joints experimentally infected with *S aureus* with either amikacin alone or amikacin combined with the optimized PL called BIOPLY.[54] Compared with amikacin alone, the amikacin + BIOPLY-treated joints had significantly decreased bacteria in synovial fluid with no detectable bacteria in 5/6 horses 7 days after treatment, decreased joint distension, synovial thickening, and fibrin on ultrasound after 7 days, shift in synovial nucleated cells from a neutrophil predominant to a monocyte predominant population, and decreases in some inflammatory mediators in synovial fluid. Of particular importance, interleukin-1 beta (IL-1β) had returned to normal preinfection concentrations by 7 days after treatment with amikacin + BIOPLY. Histologic examination of tissues at the conclusion of the study confirmed many antemortem findings with less severe fibrinosuppurative inflammation and less synovial hypertrophy, decreased inflammatory cells within the synovial membrane and greater proportion of monocytes in the amikacin + BIOPLY group. There was also decreased chondrocyte death and a dramatic reduction in proteoglycan loss in the amikacin + BIOPLY group. The results of this study are exciting and create hope for the future treatment of septic arthritis and possibly other infections with resistant biofilms.

SUMMARY

PRP continues to hold promise for treatment of musculoskeletal injuries in horses. Progress in basic science and clinical investigation has been frustratingly slow due in large part to the rapid commercialization of PRP and the seemingly insurmountable combinations of variable factors to evaluate. Only through consistent characterization of PRP products and standardization of requirements for reporting in the literature will we make progress. PL and freeze-dried PRP or platelets provide an opportunity for standardization and quality control on the PRP preparation side and could allow researchers to focus on the treatment delivery aspects of optimization. Finally, we may see the light at the end of the tunnel.

CLINICS CARE POINTS

- Equine platelet-rich plasma (PRP) often has platelet concentrations that are lower than human values for the same preparation system. Ensure the system you are using has been validated using equine blood for platelet, leukocyte, red blood cell, and growth factor concentrations.
- The volume of PRP that can be injected into tendon and ligament lesions is limited by the volume of the lesion. In one study, periligamentous injection led to visible and undesirable tissue proliferation. Limiting injection to defects in tendons or ligaments is recommended to avoid undesirable bumps.
- PRP can be kept frozen for 1 month in a −80°C freezer or 6 months in liquid nitrogen without decreases in key platelet α-granule proteins.
- Physical methods of activation such as freeze–thaw and shockwave are effective for increasing growth factor release and are less complicated than some protein or chemical methods of activation.
- The impact of nonsteroidal anti-inflammatory drugs (NSAIDs) on the effects of PRP on tissues is unknown; however, current evidence indicates that PRP quality is not impaired if it is prepared from the blood of horses already on an NSAID.
- PRP is a safe therapeutic option, with complications following injection being predominantly transient swelling and pain.

DISCLOSURE

The author has nothing to disclose.

REFERENCES

1. McCarrel TM, Mall NA, Lee AS, et al. Considerations for the use of platelet-rich plasma in orthopedics. Sports Med 2014;44(8):1025–36.
2. Fice MP, Miller JC, Christian R, et al. The Role of Platelet-Rich Plasma in Cartilage Pathology: An Updated Systematic Review of the Basic Science Evidence. Arthroscopy 2019;35(3):961–976 e963.
3. Fortier LA, Barker JU, Strauss EJ, et al. The role of growth factors in cartilage repair. Clin Orthop Relat Res 2011;469(10):2706–15.
4. Anitua E, Andia I, Ardanza B, et al. Autologous platelets as a source of proteins for healing and tissue regeneration. Thromb Haemost 2004;91(1):4–15.
5. Boswell SG, Cole BJ, Sundman EA, et al. Platelet-rich plasma: a milieu of bioactive factors. Arthroscopy 2012;28(3):429–39.
6. McCarrel TM, Minas T, Fortier LA. Optimization of leukocyte concentration in platelet-rich plasma for the treatment of tendinopathy. J Bone Joint Surg Am 2012;94(19). e143(e141-148).
7. Boswell SG, Schnabel LV, Mohammed HO, et al. Increasing platelet concentrations in leukocyte-reduced platelet-rich plasma decrease collagen gene synthesis in tendons. Am J Sports Med 2014;42(1):42–9.

8. Anitua E, Zalduendo M, Troya M, et al. Leukocyte Inclusion within a Platelet Rich Plasma-Derived Fibrin Scaffold Stimulates a More Pro-Inflammatory Environment and Alters Fibrin Properties. PLoS One 2015;10(3).
9. Anitua E, Zalduendo MM, Prado R, et al. Morphogen and proinflammatory cytokine release kinetics from PRGF-Endoret fibrin scaffolds: Evaluation of the effect of leukocyte inclusion. J Biomed Mater Res 2015;103(3):1011–20.
10. Anitua E, Sanchez M, Zalduendo MM, et al. Fibroblastic response to treatment with different preparations rich in growth factors. Cell Prolif 2009;42(2):162–70.
11. Sadoghi P, Lohberger B, Aigner B, et al. Effect of platelet-rich plasma on the biologic activity of the human rotator-cuff fibroblasts: A controlled in vitro study. J Orthop Res 2013;31(8):1249–53.
12. Dohan Ehrenfest DM, Rasmusson L, Albrektsson T. Classification of platelet concentrates: from pure platelet-rich plasma (P-PRP) to leucocyte- and platelet-rich fibrin (L-PRF). Trends Biotechnol 2009;27(3):158–67.
13. Anitua E, Padilla S, Prado R, et al. Platelet-rich plasma: are the obtaining methods, classification and clinical outcome always connected? Regen Med 2022;17(12):887–90.
14. Hessel LN, Bosch G, van Weeren PR, et al. Equine autologous platelet concentrates: A comparative study between different available systems. Equine Vet J 2015;47(3):319–25.
15. McClain AK, McCarrel TM. The effect of four different freezing conditions and time in frozen storage on the concentration of commonly measured growth factors and enzymes in equine platelet-rich plasma over six months. BMC Vet Res 2019;15(1):292.
16. Schnabel LV, Mohammed HO, Miller BJ, et al. Platelet rich plasma (PRP) enhances anabolic gene expression patterns in flexor digitorum superficialis tendons. J Orthop Res 2007;25(2):230–40.
17. Gilbertie JM, Schaer TP, Schubert AG, et al. Platelet-rich plasma lysate displays antibiofilm properties and restores antimicrobial activity against synovial fluid biofilms in vitro. J Orthop Res 2020;38(6):1365–74.
18. Pennati A, Apfelbeck T, Brounts S, et al. Washed Equine Platelet Extract as an Anti-Inflammatory Biologic Pharmaceutical. Tissue Eng Part A 2021;27(9–10):582–92.
19. Velloso Alvarez A, Boone LH, Braim AP, et al. A Survey of Clinical Usage of Non-steroidal Intra-Articular Therapeutics by Equine Practitioners. Front Vet Sci 2020;7:579967.
20. Knott LE, Fonseca-Martinez BA, O'Connor AM, et al. Current use of biologic therapies for musculoskeletal disease: A survey of board-certified equine specialists. Vet Surg 2022;51(4):557–67.
21. Schnabel LV, Sonea HO, Jacobson MS, et al. Effects of platelet rich plasma and acellular bone marrow on gene expression patterns and DNA content of equine suspensory ligament explant cultures. Equine Vet J 2008;40(3):260–5.
22. McCarrel T, Fortier L. Temporal growth factor release from platelet-rich plasma, trehalose lyophilized platelets, and bone marrow aspirate and their effect on tendon and ligament gene expression. J Orthop Res 2009;27(8):1033–42.
23. Bosch G, van Schie HT, de Groot MW, et al. Effects of platelet-rich plasma on the quality of repair of mechanically induced core lesions in equine superficial digital flexor tendons: A placebo-controlled experimental study. J Orthop Res 2010;28(2):211–7.
24. Bosch G, Moleman M, Barneveld A, et al. The effect of platelet-rich plasma on the neovascularization of surgically created equine superficial digital flexor tendon lesions. Scand J Med Sci Sports 2011;21(4):554–61.

25. Bosch G, Rene van Weeren P, Barneveld A, et al. Computerised analysis of standardised ultrasonographic images to monitor the repair of surgically created core lesions in equine superficial digital flexor tendons following treatment with intratendinous platelet rich plasma or placebo. Vet J 2011;187(1):92–8.
26. Thorpe CT, Stark RJ, Goodship AE, et al. Mechanical properties of the equine superficial digital flexor tendon relate to specific collagen cross-link levels. Equine Vet J Suppl 2010;(38):538–43.
27. Scala M, Lenarduzzi S, Spagnolo F, et al. Regenerative medicine for the treatment of Teno-desmic injuries of the equine. A series of 150 horses treated with platelet-derived growth factors. In Vivo 2014;28(6):1119–23.
28. Witte S, Dedman C, Harriss F, et al. Comparison of treatment outcomes for superficial digital flexor tendonitis in National Hunt racehorses. Vet J 2016;216:157–63.
29. Waselau M, Sutter WW, Genovese RL, et al. Intralesional injection of platelet-rich plasma followed by controlled exercise for treatment of midbody suspensory ligament desmitis in Standardbred racehorses. J Am Vet Med Assoc 2008;232(10):1515–20.
30. Garrett KS, Bramlage LR, Spike-Pierce DL, et al. Injection of platelet- and leukocyte-rich plasma at the junction of the proximal sesamoid bone and the suspensory ligament branch for treatment of yearling Thoroughbreds with proximal sesamoid bone inflammation and associated suspensory ligament branch desmitis. J Am Vet Med Assoc 2013;243(1):120–5.
31. Giunta K, Donnell JR, Donnell AD, et al. Prospective randomized comparison of platelet rich plasma to extracorporeal shockwave therapy for treatment of proximal suspensory pain in western performance horses. Res Vet Sci 2019;126:38–44.
32. Maleas G, Mageed M. Effectiveness of Platelet-Rich Plasma and Bone Marrow Aspirate Concentrate as Treatments for Chronic Hindlimb Proximal Suspensory Desmopathy. Front Vet Sci 2021;8:678453.
33. Southworth TM, Naveen NB, Tauro TM, et al. The Use of Platelet-Rich Plasma in Symptomatic Knee Osteoarthritis. J Knee Surg 2019;32(1):37–45.
34. Textor JA, Tablin F. Intra-articular use of a platelet-rich product in normal horses: clinical signs and cytologic responses. Vet Surg 2013;42(5):499–510.
35. Mirza MH, Bommala P, Richbourg HA, et al. Gait Changes Vary among Horses with Naturally Occurring Osteoarthritis Following Intra-articular Administration of Autologous Platelet-Rich Plasma. Front Vet Sci 2016;3:29.
36. Smit Y, Marais HJ, Thompson PN, et al. Clinical findings, synovial fluid cytology and growth factor concentrations after intra-articular use of a platelet-rich product in horses with osteoarthritis. J S Afr Vet Assoc 2019;90(0):e1–9.
37. De Angelis E, Grolli S, Saleri R, et al. Platelet lysate reduces the chondrocyte dedifferentiation during in vitro expansion: Implications for cartilage tissue engineering. Res Vet Sci 2020;133:98–105.
38. Perrone G, Lastra Y, González C, et al. Treatment With Platelet Lysate Inhibits Proteases of Synovial Fluid in Equines With Osteoarthritis. J Equine Vet Sci 2020;88:102952.
39. Gilbertie JM, Long JM, Schubert AG, et al. Pooled Platelet-Rich Plasma Lysate Therapy Increases Synoviocyte Proliferation and Hyaluronic Acid Production While Protecting Chondrocytes From Synoviocyte-Derived Inflammatory Mediators. Front Vet Sci 2018;5:150.
40. Garbin LC, Contino EK, Olver CS, et al. A safety evaluation of allogeneic freeze-dried platelet-rich plasma or conditioned serum compared to autologous frozen products equivalents in equine healthy joints. BMC Vet Res 2022;18(1):141.

41. Davis JG, García-López JM. Arthroscopic findings and long-term outcomes in 76 sport horses with meniscal injuries (2008-2018). Vet Surg 2022;51(3):409–17.
42. Textor JA, Tablin F. Activation of equine platelet-rich plasma: comparison of methods and characterization of equine autologous thrombin. Vet Surg 2012; 41(7):784–94.
43. Seabaugh KA, Thoresen M, Giguère S. Extracorporeal Shockwave Therapy Increases Growth Factor Release from Equine Platelet-Rich Plasma In Vitro. Front Vet Sci 2017;4:205.
44. Fukuda K, Kuroda T, Tamura N, et al. Optimal activation methods for maximizing the concentrations of platelet-derived growth factor-BB and transforming growth factor-beta 1 in equine platelet-rich plasma. J Vet Med Sci 2020;82(10):1472–9.
45. Warner TD, Nylander S, Whatling C. Anti-platelet therapy: cyclo-oxygenase inhibition and the use of aspirin with particular regard to dual anti-platelet therapy. Br J Clin Pharmacol 2011;72(4):619–33.
46. Reiter R, Resch U, Sinzinger H. Do human platelets express COX-2? Prostaglandins Leukot Essent Fatty Acids 2001;64(6):299–305.
47. Heath MF, Evans RJ, Poole AW, et al. The effects of aspirin and paracetamol on the aggregation of equine blood platelets. J Vet Pharmacol Ther 1994;17(5): 374–8.
48. Schippinger G, Pruller F, Divjak M, et al. Autologous Platelet-Rich Plasma Preparations: Influence of Nonsteroidal Anti-inflammatory Drugs on Platelet Function. Orthop J Sports Med 2015;3(6). 2325967115588896.
49. Ludwig HC, Birdwhistell KE, Brainard BM, et al. Use of a Cyclooxygenase-2 Inhibitor Does Not Inhibit Platelet Activation or Growth Factor Release From Platelet-Rich Plasma. Am J Sports Med 2017;45(14):3351–7.
50. McCarrel TM, Beatty SSK, Merrill KA, Doty A. The effect of commonly used NSAIDs on platelet function in PRP. Paper presented at: 2020 ACVS Surgery Summit; 15 September 2020, 2020; Virtual conference. The meeting was supposed to be held October 21-24, 2020 in Washington, DC.
51. Yeaman MR. The role of platelets in antimicrobial host defense. Clin Infect Dis 1997;25(5):951–68, quiz 969-970.
52. Yeaman MR, Tang YQ, Shen AJ, et al. Purification and in vitro activities of rabbit platelet microbicidal proteins. Infect Immun 1997;65(3):1023–31.
53. Aktan I, Dunkel B, Cunningham FM. Equine platelets inhibit E. coli growth and can be activated by bacterial lipopolysaccharide and lipoteichoic acid although superoxide anion production does not occur and platelet activation is not associated with enhanced production by neutrophils. Vet Immunol Immunopathol 2013;152(3–4):209–17.
54. Gilbertie JM, Schaer TP, Engiles JB, et al. A Platelet-Rich Plasma-Derived Biologic Clears *Staphylococcus aureus* Biofilms While Mitigating Cartilage Degeneration and Joint Inflammation in a Clinically Relevant Large Animal Infectious Arthritis Model. Front Cell Infect Microbiol 2022;12:895022.

Equine Autologous Conditioned Serum and Autologous Protein Solution

Kyla F. Ortved, DVM, PhD, DACVS, DACVSMR

KEYWORDS

- Orthobiologics • Regenerative medicine • Tendonitis • Desmitis • Osteoarthritis
- Joint injury

KEY POINTS

- Musculoskeletal injuries are common in equine athletes with spontaneous healing of joints, tendons, and ligaments yielding biomechanically inferior repair tissue that is prone to reinjury.
- Orthobiologics can be used to improve the quality of repair tissue.
- Autologous blood-based products, or hemoderivatives, are derived through processing of whole blood to concentrate various cytokines and growth factors.
- Autologous conditioned serum and autologous protein solution are 2 hemoderivatives used to treat joint injuries and soft tissue injuries in the horse.

INTRODUCTION

Musculoskeletal injuries involving joints, tendons, and ligaments occur commonly in the horse, especially in those performing in athletic pursuits. Such injuries present challenges, as the healing process can be difficult and time-consuming and can ultimately lead to decreased performance or retirement from sport. Articular cartilage has poor intrinsic healing capabilities largely because of its avascular nature with joint trauma often leading to secondary osteoarthritis (OA).[1,2] Although there is greater healing potential in tendons and ligaments, the healed tissue is often fibrotic, biomechanically inferior, and at risk of reinjury.[3,4] Therefore, in treating equine musculoskeletal injuries, restoration of normal biomechanical function and structure of joints and soft tissues to allow horses to perform at previous athletic levels with reduced risk of reinjury is critical.[3,5] Because the goal of regenerative medicine is to "promote self-healing through endogenous recruitment or exogenous delivery of appropriate cells, biomolecules and supporting structures,"[6] orthobiologics have been intensely investigated and used clinically in attempts to improve healing and outcomes following musculoskeletal injuries.

Clinical Studies–New Bolton Center, University of Pennsylvania, 382 West Street Road, Kennett Square, PA 19348, USA
E-mail address: kortved@vet.upenn.edu

Vet Clin Equine 39 (2023) 443–451
https://doi.org/10.1016/j.cveq.2023.07.002
vetequine.theclinics.com

Autologous blood-based products or hemoderivatives are one of the main categories of orthobiologics used in the horse. Although several different products are available, all hemoderivatives are produced by processing the patient's blood to increase concentrations of anti-inflammatory cytokines, immunomodulatory cytokines, and/or growth factors. Anti-inflammatory and immunomodulatory cytokines are desirable, as the complex inflammatory cascades that occur following injuries to joints, tendons, or ligaments are thought to drive further tissue damage and limit healing.[7–9] Growth factors are appealing, as they can promote angiogenesis, extracellular matrix (ECM) production, and tissue repair.[10–12] Following processing, the final hemoderivative product can be administered intra-articularly to treat joints or intralesionally or intrathecally to treat tendon and ligament injuries. Autologous conditioned serum (ACS) and autologous protein solution (APS) are both autologous blood-based products that are commonly used to treat joint disorders and can also be used treat tendon and ligament injuries.

AUTOLOGOUS CONDITIONED SERUM

ACS was first introduced to clinical practice as a hemoderivative with concentrated interleukin-1 receptor antagonist protein (IL-1Ra or IRAP).[13] The ability to increase endogenous production of IL-1Ra by white blood cells (WBCs) incubated in a collection device was appealing, as IL-1Ra is a competitive antagonist of IL-1α and IL-1β, both of which are proinflammatory via activation of NF-κB.[14] In joint disorders, IL-1β specifically is highly expressed by activated chondrocytes and synoviocytes and is known to be a central driver of articular inflammation with downstream effects including increased production of key degradative enzymes, matrix metalloproteinases (MMP), and a disintegrin and metalloproteinase with thrombospondin motifs (ADAMTS) or aggrecanases.[15,16] Both MMPs (MMP 1, 3, and 13) and ADAMTSs (ADAMTS-4 and -5) degrade proteoglycans and type II collagen in the ECM leading to progressive loss of cartilage function.[17] Although ACS contains concentrated IL-1Ra, further investigation into the product revealed that conditioned serum also contained high concentrations of various other anti-inflammatory and immunomodulatory factors as well as some proinflammatory cytokines, including IL-10, fibroblastic growth factor (FGF), vascular endothelial growth factor (VEGF), insulin-like growth factor-1 (IGF-1), platelet-derived growth factor (PDGF), transforming growth factor (TGF)-β, IL-1β, and tumor necrosis factor (TNF)-α.[18–20]

ACS is produced from whole blood collected under sterile conditions. Currently available systems for production of ACS include IRAP-II (Arthrex, Naples, FL, USA), IRAP ProEAS (Arthrex), and Orthokine vet irap (Dechra Veterinary Products, Overland Park, KS, USA) (**Fig. 1**). In these systems, whole blood is collected into a tube or syringe containing borosilicate beads and incubated for 24 hours at 37°C. Incubation stimulates WBCs, mainly monocytes, to produce IL-1Ra and other anti-inflammatory cytokines and growth factors. Following incubation, the tube or syringe is centrifuged to isolate the serum, which is collected into sterile syringes in preparation for injection. Because a large volume of serum is produced, extra doses can be frozen at −20°C up to 12 months for future use.[21] Since the introduction of ACS, several studies have demonstrated that incubation of blood with specialized beads is unnecessary to increase IL-1Ra production by WBCs, as the concentration of IL-1Ra increases in a time-dependent manner in glass or plastic serum separator tubes.[18,22–24] Recent studies have also investigated the development of an allogeneic, freeze-dried, off-the-shelf product in order to eliminate the need for incubation at time of patient assessment. Investigators have demonstrated that freeze-dried ACS has similar in vitro properties to fresh ACS in an OA model using stimulated cartilage explants and that freeze-dried

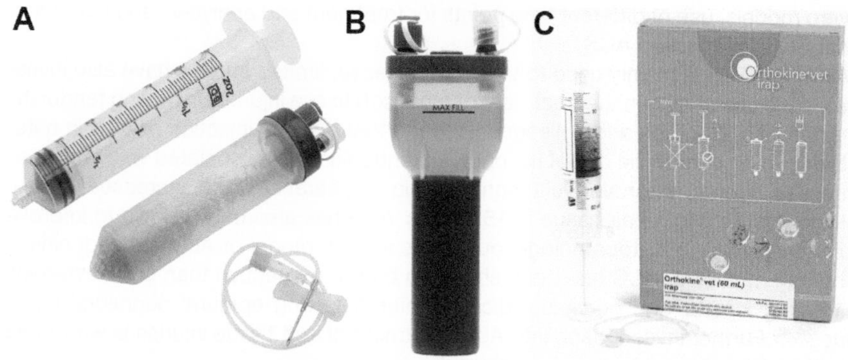

Fig. 1. ACS is commercially available from Arthrex as (*A*) IRAP-II and (*B*) IRAP ProEAS, and from Dechra Pharmaceuticals (Dechra Pharmaceuticals) as (*C*) Orthokine vet irap. Whole blood is collected or transferred into the device containing glass beads for incubation overnight. During incubation, WBCs produce IL-1Ra and other cytokines, which are concentrated in the serum after centrifugation. The conditioned serum is then injected into the affected joint or soft tissue. ([A] This image provided courtesy of Arthrex, Inc. [B] This image provided courtesy of Arthrex, Inc. [C] Orthokine® vet irap 60, with permission from ORTHOGEN Veterinary GmbH.)

products are safe for use in healthy equine joints.[25,26] Future studies examining the potential therapeutic effects of freeze-dried ACS in vivo are underway.

In addition to the effects of processing, several studies have investigated interdonor variability in ACS constituents.[18,23,27] Marques-Smith and colleauges[28] demonstrated that "responders," horses with significant improvement in lameness following ACS injection, had significantly increased concentrations of IGF-1 and IL-1Ra in their ACS when compared with "nonresponders." Investigators have also demonstrated that surgical stress[27] and strenuous exercise[29] significantly decrease IL-1Ra concentrations in equine ACS such that blood should be collected for ACS preparation before or a minimum of 24 hours after surgery or strenuous exercise. Further investigation into the effect of the individual ACS and other hemoderivatives is necessary.

Currently ACS is used predominantly to treat joint disorders, including acute inflammation, synovitis, and mild to moderate OA with typical treatment protocols suggesting 2 to 5 intra-articular injections, 7 to 10 days apart using a volume dependent on joint size.[30] The therapeutic effect of ACS in horses was first demonstrated by Frisbie and colleagues[31] in a carpal chip model of OA in which horses treated with ACS 14, 21, 28, and 35 days after carpal chip surgery had significantly decreased lameness scores compared with a saline control. Since then, several case series have been published describing the outcome of horses with naturally occurring OA following treatment with ACS. Most studies show some clinical improvement with ACS treatment; however, these studies are highly variable in terms of joints affected, severity of OA, and injection schedule, and all studies lacked a control group.[28,32–35] Randomized controlled trials have also demonstrated that ACS is effective at improving patient-reported outcome measures in human knee OA.[36–38] Interestingly, in vitro studies have yielded varied results regarding the effect of ACS on chondrocytes and cartilage explants. For example, Velloso Alvarez and colleagues[39] found that ACS treatment was more effective than triamcinolone at downregulating proinflammatory cytokines in cartilage and synovium cocultures stimulated with IL-1β, whereas Carlson and colleagues[40]and Löfgren and colleagues[41] found protective effects of ACS on inflamed chondrocyte pellets. Differences in study outcomes may be partially explained by the use of different in vitro models, use of different time points for treatment and analyses, and interdonor variability in processed ACS.

Although ACS is mainly used to treat joint disease, limited studies have also investigated the use of ACS in the treatment of other soft tissue injuries, including tendonitis and desmitis. Geburek and colleagues[42] found that a single injection of ACS in naturally occurring superficial digital flexor (SDF) tendonitis was associated with improved lameness scores, improved ultrasonographic appearance, and increased type 1 collagen content in repair tissue in 15 horses. ACS has also been shown to improve biomechanical and histopathologic outcomes in a rat model of Achilles tendonitis.[43] In human medicine, ACS has been shown to be more effective than corticosteroids at treating lumbar and cervical radiculopathies following epidural perineural injections.[44,45] Further investigation into ACS treatment of soft tissue injuries is warranted in both veterinary and human medicine.

AUTOLOGOUS PROTEIN SOLUTION

APS is produced from whole blood collected into a 60-mL syringe under sterile conditions. As the product aims to concentrate platelets and WBCs, the anticoagulant acetate citrate dextrose (ACD) is drawn up into the syringe before blood collection. APS does not require an incubation period and can be generated stall-side using a dual-device system that undergoes a two-step centrifugation process with the final product ready to inject within 20 minutes (Pro-Stride, Zoetis, Parsippany, NJ, USA) (**Fig. 2**). In the first centrifugation step, the APS separator device concentrates platelets and WBCs in a small volume of plasma. This portion of blood is then transferred to the APS concentrator device, which filters the blood through polyacrylamide beads in a second centrifugation step. The final APS product contains concentrated platelets (~3.6-fold increase), WBCs (~9-fold increase), and plasma proteins. APS is designed to combine the beneficial effects of ACS, containing concentrated amounts of IL-1Ra

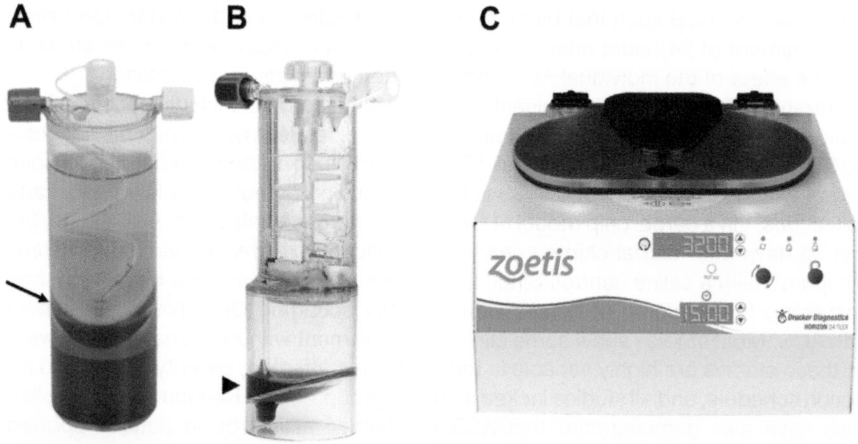

Fig. 2. APS is made using a 2-step centrifugation process. Blood is sterilely collected into a 60-mL syringe containing 5 mL of ACD and then placed into the APS separator device (*A*) for centrifugation. A small portion of blood containing concentrated platelets and WBCs (*arrow*) is then transferred to the APS concentrator device (*B*), which filters the blood through polyacrylamide beads in a second centrifugation step yielding the final product for injection (*arrowhead*). (*C*) A commercial centrifuge is required for processing. ([C] ZOETIS UNIVERSAL CENTRIFUGE, with permission from Zoetis Services LLC.)

and other anti-inflammatory cytokines produced by WBCs, with the therapeutic effects of platelet-rich plasma (PRP), containing concentrated amounts growth factors. The biologic activity of PRP is dependent on α-granule degranulation, which releases growth factors, including PDGF, TGF-β, FGF, and VEGF, that modulate the healing response of tissue.[46] A final volume of 3 to 4 mL of APS is yielded from 60 mL of blood, with treatment protocols recommending a single intra-articular injection.

Like ACS, APS has been mainly used to treat joint disorders. Several in vitro studies have sought to characterize the biologic profile and effects of APS. Woodell-May and colleagues[47] first demonstrated that human APS contained high concentrations of growth factors, including a 6.8-fold increase in PDGF-AB, a 2.7-fold increase in VEGF, and a 5.1-fold increase in epidermal growth factor when compared with whole blood. Interestingly, a recent study of human APS found that APS processing alters the lymphoid and myeloid cell populations such that, although neutrophils and T cells are the most abundant immune cell type in APS, monocytes experience the largest fold increase.[48] The investigators speculate that the alteration in WBC composition may contribute to its therapeutic effects, again supporting the effect of donor of the final product constituents. The biologic profile of the equine APS includes concentrated IL-1Ra (up to 100-fold increase) and a high IL-1Ra:IL-1β ratio (up to 1500:1) when compared with serum.[49,50] The IL-1Ra:IL-1β ratio is thought to be critical for therapeutic effects, as previous studies have demonstrated that 10 to 100 times more IL-1Ra is needed to effectively inhibit IL-1 signaling.[51] APS also contains increased amounts of soluble TNF receptor 1, IL-10, and TGF-β1.[49,50] TGF-β1 is an important anabolic factor involved in maintenance of health articular cartilage,[52,53] although it should be noted that TGF-β1 has also been reported to increase osteophyte formation and synovial fibrosis in mouse models of OA.[54,55]

The potential therapeutic effects of APS have been investigated both in vitro and in vivo. Stimulated human chondrocytes treated with APS had significantly decreased production of MMP-13,[47] whereas APS-treated equine chondrocyte cultures contained significantly increased amounts of IL-1Ra and IL-10,[49] both of which are chondroprotective.[56–60] APS-treated cultures also contained increased concentrations of IL-6,[49] a modulatory cytokine that can support chondrocyte homeostasis.[61,62] Bertone and colleagues[50] investigated the effects of a single intra-articular APS injection in horses with naturally occurring OA. The investigators demonstrated that horses treated with APS ($n = 20$) had significantly improved lameness scores, decreased asymmetry in vertical peak forces, and increased range of motion of affected joints 14 days after treatment when compared with horses in the saline-treated control group ($n = 20$). In addition, client-reported lameness remained improved at 3 and 12 months after APS treatment when compared with baseline. APS has also been shown to improve clinical signs associated with knee OA in human patients[63,64] and in dogs with OA.[65]

Treatment of tendon and ligament injuries with APS has not been widely reported in the literature but is in use in clinical practice.[30] In one experimental study examining the effects of APS on healing of collagenase-induced SDF tendonitis, decreased expression of collagen type III was noted in APS-treated tendons versus saline-treated control tendons. Collagen type III is thought to be undesirable, as it has less elasticity than collagen type I, resulting in inferior biomechanical healing.[43,66] In addition, APS-treated tendons had a higher elastic modulus than saline-treated tendon, and although the investigators report the difference was not statistically significant, the increase (103 MPa in APS-treated vs 80 MPa in saline-treated) could be clinically relevant. In a study by Geburek and colleagues,[66] normal equine tendon was reported to have an elastic modulus of 175 MPa. The use of APS to treat soft tissue injuries in horses and other species requires further investigation.

SUMMARY

Orthobiologics can improve healing and clinical outcomes owing to their anti-inflammatory, immunomodulatory, and anabolic properties, all which support tissue healing and restoration of normal structure and function. Autologous blood-based products, including ACS and APS, are easily accessible and simple to produce. In vitro and in vivo evidence supports the use of both hemoderivatives in the treatment of joint disease and soft tissue injuries; however, further research is needed to optimize treatment protocols and outcomes. In addition, greater understanding of interdonor variability and the potential impact on therapeutic benefits is needed.

DISCLOSURE

The author declares no conflict of interest related to this report.

REFERENCES

1. Mankin HJ. The response of articular cartilage to mechanical injury. J Bone Jt Surgery American 1982;64(3):460–6.
2. Strauss EJ, Goodrich LR, Chen CT, et al. Biochemical and biomechanical properties of lesion and adjacent articular cartilage after chondral defect repair in an equine model. Am J Sports Med 2005;33(11):1647–53.
3. Dyson SJ. Medical management of superficial digital flexor tendonitis: a comparative study in 219 horses (1992-2000). Equine Vet J 2004;36(5):415–9.
4. O'meara B, Bladon B, Parkin TDH, et al. An investigation of the relationship between race performance and superficial digital flexor tendonitis in the Thoroughbred racehorse. Equine Vet J 2010;42(4):322–6.
5. Dyson S. Proximal suspensory desmitis in the hindlimb: 42 cases. Br Vet J 1994;150(3):279–91.
6. Advancing tissue science and engineering: a foundation for the future. A multiagency strategic plan. Tissue Eng 2007;13(12):2825–6.
7. Benito MJ, Veale DJ, FitzGerald O, et al. Synovial tissue inflammation in early and late osteoarthritis. Ann Rheum Dis 2005;64(9):1263–7.
8. Goldring MB, Otero M. Inflammation in osteoarthritis. Curr Opin Rheumatol 2011;23(5):471–8.
9. Fredberg U, Stengaard-Pedersen K. Chronic tendinopathy tissue pathology, pain mechanisms, and etiology with a special focus on inflammation. Scand J Med Sci Sports 2008;18(1):3–15.
10. Chan BP, Fu SC, Qin L, et al. Supplementation-time dependence of growth factors in promoting tendon healing. Clin Orthop Relat Res 2006;448:240–7.
11. Ortved KF, Begum L, Mohammed HO, et al. Implantation of rAAV5-IGF-I transduced autologous chondrocytes improves cartilage repair in full-thickness defects in the equine model. Mol Ther 2015;23(2):363–73.
12. Goodrich LR, Hidaka C, Robbins PD, et al. Genetic modification of chondrocytes with insulin-like growth factor-1 enhances cartilage healing in an equine model. J Bone Jt Surgery British 2007;89(5):672–85.
13. Meijer H, Reinecke J, Becker C, et al. The production of anti-inflammatory cytokines in whole blood by physico-chemical induction. Inflamm Res 2003;52(10):404–7.
14. Granowitz EV, Clark BD, Mancilla J, et al. Interleukin-1 receptor antagonist competitively inhibits the binding of interleukin-1 to the type II interleukin-1 receptor. J Biol Chem 1991;266(22):14147–50.

15. Goldring MB, Berenbaum F. The regulation of chondrocyte function by proinflammatory mediators: prostaglandins and nitric oxide. Clin Orthop Relat Res 2004; 427(Suppl):S37–46.
16. Kamm JL, Nixon AJ, Witte TH. Cytokine and catabolic enzyme expression in synovium, synovial fluid and articular cartilage of naturally osteoarthritic equine carpi. Equine Vet J 2010;42(8):693–9.
17. Little CB, Flannery CR, Hughes CE, et al. Aggrecanase versus matrix metalloproteinases in the catabolism of the interglobular domain of aggrecan in vitro. Biochem J 1999;344 Pt(1):61–8.
18. Hraha TH, Doremus KM, Mcilwraith CW, et al. Autologous conditioned serum: the comparative cytokine profiles of two commercial methods (IRAP and IRAP II) using equine blood. Equine Vet J 2011;43(5):516–21 [doi].
19. Rutgers M, Saris DB, Dhert WJ, et al. Cytokine profile of autologous conditioned serum for treatment of osteoarthritis, in vitro effects on cartilage metabolism and intra-articular levels after injection. Arthritis Res Ther 2010;12(3):R114.
20. Wehling P, Moser C, Frisbie D, et al. Autologous conditioned serum in the treatment of orthopedic diseases: the orthokine therapy. BioDrugs 2007;21(5):323–32.
21. Barreto A, Braun TR. A method to induce interleukin-1 receptor antagonist protein from autologous whole blood. Cytokine 2016;81:137–41.
22. Hale J, Hughes K, Hall S, et al. Effects of production method and repeated freeze thaw cycles on cytokine concentrations and microbial contamination in equine autologous conditioned serum. Front Vet Sci 2021;8:759828.
23. Lasarzik de Ascurra J, Ehrle A, Einspanier R, et al. Influence of incubation time and incubation tube on the cytokine and growth factor concentrations of autologous conditioned serum in horses. J Equine Vet Sci 2019;75:30–4.
24. Nakken G, Kirk J, Fjordbakk CT. Cytokine enrichment in equine conditioned serum is not reliant on incubation in specialized containers. Vet Immunol Immunopathol 2023;258:110576.
25. Garbin LC, Contino EK, Olver CS, et al. A safety evaluation of allogeneic freeze-dried platelet-rich plasma or conditioned serum compared to autologous frozen products equivalents in equine healthy joints. BMC Vet Res 2022;18(1):141.
26. Garbin LC, McIlwraith CW, Frisbie DD. Use of allogeneic freeze-dried conditioned serum for the prevention of degradation in cartilage exposed to IL-1ß. BMC Vet Res 2022;18(1):265.
27. Fjordbakk CT, Johansen GM, Løvås AC, et al. Surgical stress influences cytokine content in autologous conditioned serum. Equine Vet J 2015;47(2):212–7.
28. Marques-Smith P, Kallerud AS, Johansen GM, et al. Is clinical effect of autologous conditioned serum in spontaneously occurring equine articular lameness related to ACS cytokine profile? BMC Vet Res 2020;16(1):181.
29. Hale JN, Hughes KJ, Hall S, et al. The effect of exercise on cytokine concentration in equine autologous conditioned serum. Equine Vet J 2023;55(3):551–6.
30. Knott LE, Fonseca-Martinez BA, O'Connor AM, et al. Current use of biologic therapies for musculoskeletal disease: a survey of board-certified equine specialists. Vet Surg 2022;51(4):557–67.
31. Frisbie DD, Kawcak CE, Werpy NM, et al. Clinical, biochemical, and histologic effects of intra-articular administration of autologous conditioned serum in horses with experimentally induced osteoarthritis. Am J Vet Res 2007;68(3):290–6.
32. Chiaradia E, Pepe M, Tartaglia M, et al. Gambling on putative biomarkers of osteoarthritis and osteochondrosis by equine synovial fluid proteomics. J Proteomics 2012;75(14):4478–93.

33. Lasarzik J, Bondzio A, Rettig M, et al. Evaluation of two protocols using autologous conditioned serum for intra-articular therapy of equine osteoarthritis—A pilot study monitoring cytokines and cartilage-specific biomarkers. J Equine Vet Sci 2018;60:35–42.
34. Schneider U, Veith G. First results on the outcome of gold-induced, autologous conditioned serum (GOLDIC) in the treatment of different lameness-associated equine diseases. J Cell Sci Ther 2013;5(1):151–6.
35. Warner K, Schulze T, Lischer C. Behandlung von osteoarthritis mit ACS (IRAP®) bei 26 pferdon - Retrospektive studie. PFERDEHEILKUNDE 2016;32(3):241–8.
36. Yang KGA, Raijmakers NJH, van Arkel ERA, et al. Autologous interleukin-1 receptor antagonist improves function and symptoms in osteoarthritis when compared to placebo in a prospective randomized controlled trial. Osteoarthritis Cartilage 2008;16(4):498–505.
37. Baltzer AWA, Moser C, Jansen SA, et al. Autologous conditioned serum (Orthokine) is an effective treatment for knee osteoarthritis. Osteoarthritis Cartilage 2009;17(2):152–60.
38. Raeissadat SA, Rayegani SM, Sohrabi MR, et al. Effectiveness of intra-articular autologous-conditioned serum injection in knee osteoarthritis: a meta-analysis study. Futur Sci OA 2021;7(9):FSO759.
39. Velloso Alvarez A, Boone LH, Pondugula SR, et al. Effects of autologous conditioned serum, autologous protein solution, and triamcinolone on inflammatory and catabolic gene expression in equine cartilage and synovial explants treated with IL-1β in co-culture. Front Vet Sci 2020;7:323.
40. Carlson ER, Stewart AA, Carlson KL, et al. Effects of serum and autologous conditioned serum on equine articular chondrocytes treated with interleukin-1β. Am J Vet Res 2013;74(5):700–5.
41. Löfgren M, Ekman S, Ekholm J, et al. Conditioned serum in vitro treatment of chondrocyte pellets and osteoarthritic explants. Equine Vet J 2023;55(2):325–35.
42. Geburek F, Lietzau M, Beineke A, et al. Effect of a single injection of autologous conditioned serum (ACS) on tendon healing in equine naturally occurring tendinopathies. Stem Cell Res Ther 2015;6(1):126.
43. Genç E, Beytemur O, Yuksel S, et al. Investigation of the biomechanical and histopathological effects of autologous conditioned serum on healing of Achilles tendon. Acta Orthop Traumatol Turcica 2018;52(3):226–31.
44. Becker C, Heidersdorf S, Drewlo S, et al. Efficacy of epidural perineural injections with autologous conditioned serum for lumbar radicular compression: an investigator-initiated, prospective, double-blind, reference-controlled study. Spine 2007;32(17):1803–8.
45. Goni VG, Singh Jhala S, Gopinathan NR, et al. Efficacy of epidural perineural injection of autologous conditioned serum in unilateral cervical radiculopathy: a pilot study. Spine 2015;40(16):E915–21.
46. Boswell SG, Cole BJ, Sundman EA, et al. Platelet-rich plasma: a milieu of bioactive factors. Arthrosc J Arthrosc Relat Surg 2012;28(3):429–39.
47. Woodell-May J, Matuska A, Oyster M, et al. Autologous protein solution inhibits MMP-13 production by IL-1β and TNFα-stimulated human articular chondrocytes. J Orthop Res 2011;29(9):1320–6.
48. Peña AN, Sommerfeld SD, Anderson AE, et al. Autologous protein solution processing alters lymphoid and myeloid cell populations and modulates gene expression dependent on cell type. Arthritis Res Ther 2022;24(1):221.
49. Linardi RL, Dodson ME, Moss KL, et al. The effect of autologous protein solution on the inflammatory cascade in stimulated equine chondrocytes. Front Vet Sci 2019;6:64.

50. Bertone AL, Ishihara A, Zekas LJ, et al. Evaluation of a single intra-articular injection of autologous protein solution for treatment of osteoarthritis in horses. Am J Vet Res 2014;75(2):141–51.
51. Arend WP. Interleukin 1 receptor antagonist. A new member of the interleukin 1 family. J Clin Invest 1991;88(5):1445–51.
52. Finnson KW, Chi Y, Bou-Gharios G, et al. TGF-b signaling in cartilage homeostasis and osteoarthritis. Front Biosci (Schol Ed) 2012;4:251–68.
53. Ongchai S, Somnoo O, Kongdang P, et al. TGF-β1 upregulates the expression of hyaluronan synthase 2 and hyaluronan synthesis in culture models of equine articular chondrocytes. J Vet Sci 2018;19(6):735.
54. Blaney Davidson EN, Vitters EL, van den Berg WB, et al. TGF beta-induced cartilage repair is maintained but fibrosis is blocked in the presence of Smad7. Arthritis Res Ther 2006;8(3):R65.
55. Bakker AC, van de Loo FA, van Beuningen HM, et al. Overexpression of active TGF-beta-1 in the murine knee joint: evidence for synovial-layer-dependent chondro-osteophyte formation. Osteoarthritis Cartilage 2001;9(2):128–36.
56. Haupt JL, Frisbie DD, McIlwraith CW, et al. Dual transduction of insulin-like growth factor-I and interleukin-1 receptor antagonist protein controls cartilage degradation in an osteoarthritic culture model. J Orthop Res 2005;23(1):118–26.
57. Finnegan A, Kaplan CD, Cao Y, et al. Collagen-induced arthritis is exacerbated in IL-10-deficient mice. Arthritis Res Ther 2003;5(1):R18–24.
58. Cuzzocrea S, Mazzon E, Dugo L, et al. Absence of endogeneous interleukin-10 enhances the evolution of murine type-II collagen-induced arthritis. Eur Cytokine Netw 2001;12(4):568–80.
59. Ortved KF, Begum L, Stefanovski D, et al. AAV-mediated overexpression of IL-10 mitigates the inflammatory cascade in stimulated equine chondrocyte pellets. Curr Gene Ther 2018;18(3):171–9.
60. Frisbie DD, Ghivizzani SC, Robbins PD, et al. Treatment of experimental equine osteoarthritis by in vivo delivery of the equine interleukin-1 receptor antagonist gene. Gene Ther 2002;9(1):12–20.
61. Ley C, Svala E, Nilton A, et al. Effects of high mobility group box protein-1, interleukin-1β, and interleukin-6 on cartilage matrix metabolism in three-dimensional equine chondrocyte cultures. Connect Tissue Res 2011;52(4):290–300.
62. Svala E, Thorfve AI, Ley C, et al. Effects of interleukin-6 and interleukin-1β on expression of growth differentiation factor-5 and Wnt signaling pathway genes in equine chondrocytes. Am J Vet Res 2014;75(2):132–40.
63. Hix J, Klaassen M, Foreman R, et al. An autologous anti-Inflammatory protein solution yielded a favorable safety profile and significant pain relief in an open-label pilot study of patients with osteoarthritis. Biores Open Access 2017;6(1):151–8.
64. van Drumpt RAM, van der Weegen W, King W, et al. Safety and treatment effectiveness of a single autologous protein solution injection in patients with knee osteoarthritis. Biores Open Access 2016;5(1):261–8.
65. Wanstrath AW, Hettlich BF, Su L, et al. Evaluation of a single intra-articular injection of autologous protein solution for treatment of osteoarthritis in a canine population. Vet Surg 2016;45(6):764–74.
66. Geburek F, Roggel F, van Schie HTM, et al. Effect of single intralesional treatment of surgically induced equine superficial digital flexor tendon core lesions with adipose-derived mesenchymal stromal cells: a controlled experimental trial. Stem Cell Res Ther 2017;8(1):129.

Equine Bone Marrow Aspirate Concentrate

Lisa A. Fortier, DVM, PhD, DACVS*

KEYWORDS

• Bone marrow concentrate • BMAC • Bone marrow • cBMA • Equine

KEY POINTS

- Bone marrow concentrate is a source of autologous anabolic molecules, mesenchymal stromal cells, and a scaffold.
- Bone marrow concentrate contains supraphysiologic concentrations of interleukin-1 receptor antagonist protein and mesenchymal stromal cells; setting it apart from other biologics.
- Osteoarthritis, desmitis, and articular cartilage or bone defects are appropriate disease states for application of bone marrow concentrate.

INTRODUCTION

Bone marrow aspirate concentrate (BMC) is unique among the various biologics in regenerative medicine because it fulfills the biological triad of tissue engineering by providing cells, biophysical and chemical signals, and a scaffold (**Fig. 1**). In the musculoskeletal field, bone marrow aspirate (BMA) was first used to treat knee pain in humans.[1] Bone marrow concentrate for autologous tissue regeneration was developed in the horse nearly 15 years ago and reported in an equine model of cartilage repair.[2] Since that time, its use has expanded in clinical scope beyond the articular joint. Despite its widespread use, uncovering the mechanisms through which BMC imparts its beneficial effects on injuries remains a topic of ongoing research.

GENERATION OF BMC

Bone marrow concentrate is prepared patient-side by centrifugation of BMA. Typically, 30 to 60 mL of anticoagulated BMA (heparin or ACD-A) is filtered to remove potential bone particulate matter and then centrifuged in a commercial disposable device or in laboratory tubes to isolate the buffy coat which contains a concentrate of mesenchymal stromal cells (MSCs), leukocytes (neutrophils, lymphocytes, and monocytes), and platelets[2,3] compared to the starting BMA. Use of a commercial

Clinical Sciences, Cornell University College of Veterinary Medicine, Ithaca, NY, USA
* Corresponding author. 1931 North Meacham Road, Suite 100, Schaumburg, IL 60173-4360.
E-mail address: lfortier@avma.org

Vet Clin Equine 39 (2023) 453–459
https://doi.org/10.1016/j.cveq.2023.05.002

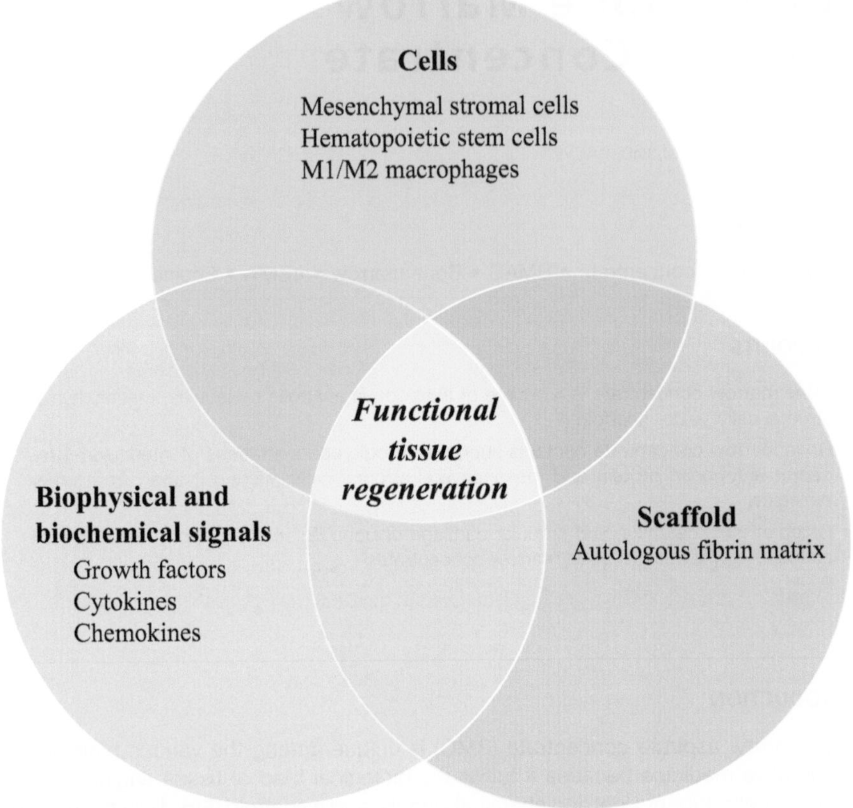

Fig. 1. Bone marrow concentrate is unique among all biologics because it provides a combination of autologous cells, biophysical and biochemical signals, and a scaffold to effectuate functional tissue regeneration.

disposable device is more convenient and can be done in the field as opposed to processing of tubes in a laboratory, and disposable devices are closed systems which minimize the potential for contamination. A gravitational filtration system has also been described as a method to concentrate BMA.[4] While this would be even more convenient than a commercial centrifugation system, it does not concentrate MSCs or platelets to the same extent as centrifugation devices.

THE CELLS IN BMC

In a more than 20-year-old, but still often-referenced manuscript by Pittenger and colleagues,[5] the quantity of MSCs in BMC is stated to be as low as 0.001% to 0.01% of the entire nucleated cell population. This led some to suggest that BMC was not a source of MSC. However, that line of thinking is consistent with the old paradigm of MSCs, when it was thought that MSCs differentiated into cells of a tissue type, thereby effectuating tissue repair. For example, to facilitate cartilage repair, it was once thought that the MSCs in BMC would differentiate into chondrocytes and become functioning resident tissue cells. It is now commonly accepted that MSCs function to effectuate repair through numerous paracrine signaling exchanges with the local

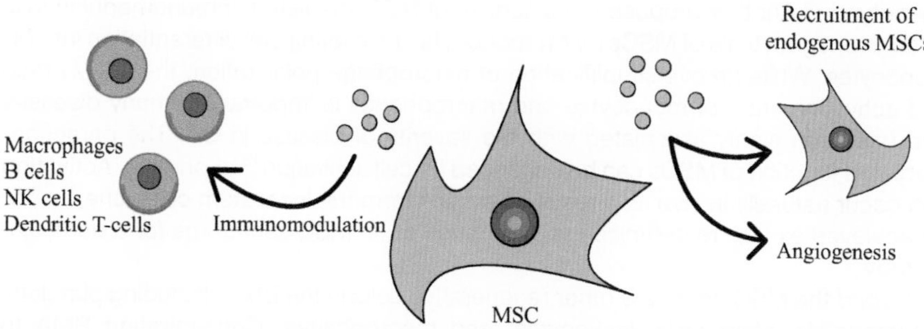

Fig. 2. The mechanism of action of mesenchymal stromal cells is thought to be through the secretome. The secretome is a milieu of trophic factors and immunomodulatory cytokines that promote functional changes in immune cells resulting in immunomodulation, recruitment of endogenous MSCs, and angiogenesis.

environment. This paracrine effect of MSCs has been observed in the laboratory since the 1970s in hematopoietic stem cells and is now commonly accepted as the mechanism of action of MSCs.[6] Because the concentration of MSCs in BMC is low, it is therefore difficult to accurately quantify with only one publication identifying MSCs using multicolor flow cytometry for simultaneous measurement of validated cell surface marker. A more simplified flow cytometry protocol for $CD45^{low}CD271^{high}$ cells has been reported as a method for quantifying MSC in BMC.[7] Even more simple to perform in the laboratory are colony-forming unit assays, which have been used as a surrogate marker for MSC in BMC, but there is no meaningful correlation between colony-forming units and MSC in BMC.[8,9] With the contemporary understanding of the immunomodulatory function of MSCs and that both MSC secretome and BMC can recruit MSCs,[10] the literal quantity of MSCs in BMC is unlikely of significant consequence. More concerning for consistent quality of repair is donor and site variability. Of note in the horse, BMA from the tuber coxae is possible, and in younger horses (2–5 years of age), it is equivalent in the yield of MSC compared to BMA from the sternum.[11] However, in older horses (13 years), a tuber coxae aspirate contains significantly less MSC than one from the sternum, which should be taken into consideration when treating mature athletes.[12] Further optimization of MSC in BMA for patient-side generation of BMC can be obtained by advancing the needle 5 mm 3 times during aspiration from each sternebrae.[13] When using the sternum, the optimal safe location for insertion of the needle has been identified as the 4–6th sternebrae using ultrasound guidance.[14]

BIOPHYSICAL AND BIOCHEMICAL SIGNALS

Like all biologics, including platelet-rich plasma (PRP), autologous conditioned serum, autologous protein solution, amnion products, and others, BMC contains both anabolic/anti-inflammatory/immunomodulatory and catabolic/proinflammatory chemokines and cytokines. The MSCs in BMC exert their paracrine reparative effects through the secretion of immunomodulatory cytokines and chemokines, collectively known as the secretome. The collective secretome promotes functional changes in monocytes/macrophages, dendritic cells, T cells, B cells, and natural killer cells and culminating in immunomodulation, recruitment of endogenous MSCs, and angiogenesis (**Fig. 2**). For example, MSC-secreted interleukin-1 receptor antagonist protein (IL-1RA, IRAP), which is a component of the MSC secretome, has been shown to enhance polarization of macrophages toward the M_2, anti-inflammatory and tissue reparative phenotype.[15] Another proposed mechanism of MSC-mediated immunomodulation is through phagocytosis of MSCs by M_1 monocytes promoting cell differentiation into M_2 monocytes. While an oversimplification of macrophage polarization, the M_1/M_2 ratio and activation state of monocytes and macrophages is important in many diseases and has been highly associated with the severity of disease in OA. The paracrine-mediated function of MSCs can be enhanced by cell activation[16] or priming. Activation can occur naturally in vivo as a result of signals from the local stem cell niche,[17,18] or be achieved ex vivo to optimize the generation of an MSC secretome for a particular therapy.

Beyond the MSC, there are other regenerative cells in the BMC, including platelets, hematopoietic stem cells, leukocytes, and macrophages. Concentrating BMA to generate cBMA results in significant increases in multiple anabolic factors, including TGF-B1, PDGF, VEGF, MCSF, VCAM-1, and IL-1RA (IRAP).[19–22] As previously stated, biologics also contain catabolic factors and those reported in BMC include IL-1B and IL-8.[19,20] It is likely that this combination of biological cues from the MSC, chemokines, and cytokines enhances tissue healing.

CLINICAL APPLICATIONS OF BMC

The clinical use of BMC for soft tissue musculoskeletal injuries in horses is not as commonly reported as it is in human patients. This might be in part due to an unsubstantiated concern that BMC could result in soft tissue mineralization, which has not been documented in equine or human patients. There is reasonable in vitro and equine patient evidence to support its use for suspensory desmopathy. In tissue culture experiments from 2 separate laboratory groups, acellular bone marrow stimulated matrix synthesis in suspensory ligament explant cultures to a greater extent than PRP.[23,24] In a clinical study of horses with chronic (>3 months) duration of proximal suspensory desmopathy in hindlimbs, 25 horses were treated with intralesional BMC, 46 with intralesional leukocyte rich platelet-rich plasma (LR-PRP), and 22 underwent controlled exercise rehabilitation without any intralesional injections.[3] Follow-up was a minimum of 18 months. Both BMC and LR-PRP were superior to the controlled exercise group with respect to resolution of the lesion of ultrasound and return to sound performance, with the BMC group having better lameness scores than the LR-PRP. Intralesional BMA (not BMC) in combination with superior check desmotomy was also found to increase the likelihood of thoroughbred racehorses to return to racing than conservative treatment.[25]

Generation and application of BMC for use in the musculoskeletal system was first developed in the horse for articular cartilage repair.[2] Injection of BMC with thrombin creates a fibrin clot as a biologic scaffold containing the increased concentration of MSCs and bioactive chemokines and cytokines to enhance tissue repair, as discussed previously. Large (15 mm diameter) full-thickness cartilage lesions were created on the lateral trochlear ridge of the femora in 12 horses. With each animal serving as its own control, one defect was filled with BMC and the other was treated with microfracture, representing the standard of care in cartilage repair. Cartilage repair with BMC resulted in increased fill of the defects, improved integration of repair tissue into surrounding normal cartilage, and improved type-II collagen and glycosaminoglycan content compared to microfracture-treated defects. The use of BMC to enhance cartilage repair, particularly to enhance the integration of osteochondral allografts or autographs, is now commonly reported in the human literature.[26,27] In the horse, BMC is most commonly used as a graft with or without debridement in cystic lesions of the medial femoral condyle, humerus, and other locations (**Fig. 3**).[28]

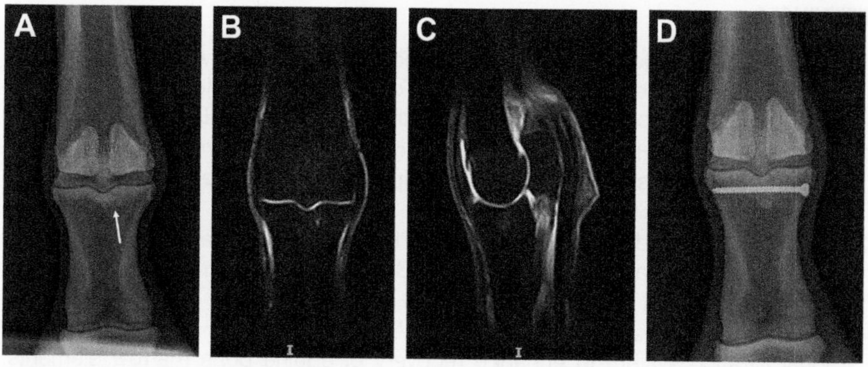

Fig. 3. (*A*) Dorsopalmar radiograph of a chronic fracture (*arrow*) in the parasagittal groove of the proximal first phalanx. MRI revealed increased STIR signal in the (*B*) dorsopalmar and (*C*) lateromedial planes delineating the extent of the fracture signal. (*D*) Using fluoroscopic guidance, a 3.5 mm self-tapping cortical bone screw was placed to stabilize the fracture, and drilling (osteostixis) of the fracture site at 3 sites was performed above the screw with a 2-0 mm drill bit followed by bone marrow concentrate administration into the drill hole and into the metacarpophalangeal joint to facilitate articular cartilage and bone repair.

SUMMARY

The generation of BMC requires a bit more technical expertise and time to obtain the BMA compared to obtaining blood to generate PRP, but otherwise the equipment required to generate either biologic is similar. However, the presence of MSC, IL-1RA, and increased anabolic growth factors in BMC compared to PRP should also be considered when choosing the optimal biologic for the patient. Clinical application of BMC should be considered for enhanced cartilage defect repair, alleviation of symptomatic osteoarthritis, bone regeneration particularly in cystic lesions, and suspensory desmitis.

CLINICS CARE POINTS

- Aspiration of BMA from the tuber coxae should be restricted to horses 3 years of age or less. The sternum is the site of choice for BMA aspiration otherwise.
- BMC provides all 3 components desired for tissue regeneration, including a scaffold, cells, and bioactive signals.
- Intralesional injection of BMC into the suspensory ligament enhances functional tissue regeneration without evidence of soft tissue mineralization.
- Bone regeneration in cystic lesions is enhanced by BMC.

DISCLOSURE

L.A. Fortier is Editor-in-Chief for the Journal of the American Veterinary Medical Association and the American Journal of Veterinary Research. Fortier is also a consultant for Arthrex, Inc.

ACKNOWLEDGMENTS

The author acknowledge the contribution of Nicole Nixon in concept, writing, editing, and generation of the contained schamtics while writing this article.

REFERENCES

1. Hauser RA, Orlofsky A. Regenerative injection therapy with whole bone marrow aspirate for degenerative joint disease: a case series. Clin Med Insights Arthritis Musculoskelet Disord 2013;6. https://doi.org/10.4137/CMAMD.S10951.
2. Fortier LA, Potter HG, Rickey EJ, et al. Concentrated bone marrow aspirate improves full-thickness cartilage repair compared with microfracture in the equine model. J Bone Jt Surg 2010;92(10):1927–37.
3. Maleas G, Mageed M. Effectiveness of Platelet-Rich Plasma and Bone Marrow Aspirate Concentrate as Treatments for Chronic Hindlimb Proximal Suspensory Desmopathy. Front Vet Sci 2021;8:673.
4. Mundy LN, Ishihara A, Wellman ML, et al. Evaluation of the ability of a gravitational filtration system to enhance recovery of equine bone marrow elements. Am J Vet Res 2015;76(6):561–9.
5. Pittenger MF, Mackay AM, Beck SC, et al. Multilineage potential of adult human mesenchymal stem cells. Science 1999;284(5411):143–7.
6. Fortier LA, Lintz M. Basic Science of Resident Stem Cells. Oper Tech Sports Med 2020;28(4):150776.
7. El-Jawhari JJ, Cuthbert R, McGonagle D, et al. The CD45lowCD271high Cell Prevalence in Bone Marrow Samples May Provide a Useful Measurement of the Bone Marrow Quality for Cartilage and Bone Regenerative Therapy. J Bone Jt Surg - Am 2017;99(15):1305–13.
8. Gaul F, Bugbee W, Cartilage HHJ-. A review of commercially available point-of-care devices to concentrate bone marrow for the treatment of osteoarthritis and focal cartilage lesions. Cartilage 2019;10(4):387–94.
9. Cercone M, Greenfield MR, Fortier LA. Bone Marrow Concentrate Mesenchymal Stromal Cells Do not Correlate With Nucleated Cell Count or Colony Forming Units. J Cartil Jt Preserv 2021;1(3):100017.
10. Holmes HL, Wilson B, Goerger JP, et al. Facilitated recruitment of mesenchymal stromal cells by bone marrow concentrate and platelet rich plasma. PLoS One 2018;13(3). https://doi.org/10.1371/JOURNAL.PONE.0194567.
11. Adams MK, Goodrich LR, Rao S, et al. Equine bone marrow-derived mesenchymal stromal cells (BMDMSCs) from the ilium and sternum: Are there differences? Equine Vet J 2013;45(3):372–5.
12. Delling U, Lindner K, Ribitsch I, et al. Comparison of bone marrow aspiration at the sternum and the tuber coxae in middle-aged horses. Can J Vet Res 2012; 76(1):52–6. Available at: https://www.ingentaconnect.com/content/cvma/cjvr/2012/00000076/00000001/art00008. Accessed January 30, 2023.
13. Peters AE, Watts AE. Biopsy needle advancement during bone marrow aspiration increases mesenchymal stem cell concentration. Front Vet Sci 2016;3:23.
14. Kasashima Y, Ueno T, Tomita A, et al. Optimisation of bone marrow aspiration from the equine sternum for the safe recovery of mesenchymal stem cells. Equine Vet J 2011;43(3):288–94.
15. Luz-Crawford P, Djouad F, Toupet K, et al. Mesenchymal Stem Cell-Derived Interleukin 1 Receptor Antagonist Promotes Macrophage Polarization and Inhibits B Cell Differentiation. Stem Cell 2016;34(2):483–92.
16. Cassano JM, Schnabel LV, Goodale MB, et al. Inflammatory licensed equine MSCs are chondroprotective and exhibit enhanced immunomodulation in an inflammatory environment. Stem Cell Res Ther 2018;9(1). https://doi.org/10.1186/S13287-018-0840-2.

17. Cassano JM, Schnabel LV, Goodale MB, et al. The immunomodulatory function of equine MSCs is enhanced by priming through an inflammatory microenvironment or TLR3 ligand. Vet Immunol Immunopathol 2018;195:33–9.
18. Kadle RL, Abdou SA, Villarreal-Ponce AP, et al. Microenvironmental cues enhance mesenchymal stem cell-mediated immunomodulation and regulatory T-cell expansion. PLoS One 2018;13(3). https://doi.org/10.1371/JOURNAL.PONE.0193178.
19. McCarrel T, Research LF-J of O. Temporal growth factor release from platelet-rich plasma, trehalose lyophilized platelets, and bone marrow aspirate and their effect on tendon and ligament gene. Wiley Online Libr 2009;27(8):1033–42.
20. Schäfer R, Debaun MR, Fleck E, et al. Quantitation of progenitor cell populations and growth factors after bone marrow aspirate concentration. J Transl Med 2019;17(1). https://doi.org/10.1186/S12967-019-1866-7.
21. Cassano JM, Kennedy JG, Ross KA, et al. Bone marrow concentrate and platelet-rich plasma differ in cell distribution and interleukin 1 receptor antagonist protein concentration. Knee Surg Sports Traumatol Arthrosc 2018;26(1):333–42.
22. Commins J, Irwin R, Matuska A, et al. Biological mechanisms for cartilage repair using a BioCartilage scaffold: Cellular adhesion/migration and bioactive proteins. Cartilage 2021;13(1_suppl):984S–92S.
23. Schnabel LV, Mohammed HO, Jacobson MS, et al. Effects of platelet rich plasma and acellular bone marrow on gene expression patterns and DNA content of equine suspensory ligament explant cultures. Equine Vet J 2008;40(3):260–5.
24. Smith JJ, Ross MW, Smith RKW. Anabolic effects of acellular bone marrow, platelet rich plasma, and serum on equine suspensory ligament fibroblasts in vitro. Vet Comp Orthop Traumatol 2006;19(1):43–7.
25. Murphy DJ, Kö-Peternelj V, Aleri JW. Intralesional bone marrow and superior check desmotomy is superior to conservative treatment of equine superficial digital flexor tendonitis. Equine Vet J 2022;54(6):1047–54.
26. Chona DV, Kha ST, Minetos PD, et al. Biologic augmentation for the operative treatment of osteochondral defects of the knee: a systematic review. Orthop J Sports Med 2021;9(11). https://doi.org/10.1177/23259671211049756.
27. Baumann CA, Baumann JR, Bozynski CC, et al. Comparison of Techniques for Preimplantation Treatment of Osteochondral Allograft Bone. J Knee Surg 2019;32(1):97–104.
28. D'Amato RD, Memeo A, Fusini F, et al. Treatment of simple bone cyst with bone marrow concentrate and equine-derived demineralized bone matrix injection versus methylprednisolone acetate injections: A retrospective comparative study. Acta Orthop Traumatol Turc 2020;54(1):49–58.

Overview of Equine Stem Cells

Sources, Practices, and Potential Safety Concerns

Thomas G. Koch, DVM, PhD*, Alexander G. Kuzma-Hunt, BSc, Keith A. Russell, PhD

KEYWORDS

• Equine • Therapy • Mesenchymal • iPSC • Clinical applications
• Tissue engineering • Pluripotent • Regenerative medicine

KEY POINTS

- Various stem cell types, including pluripotent and mesenchymal stromal/stem cells, or stem cell-derived products, may be used to treat a wide range of conditions.
- Equine stem cells may best target clinical disorders that require cell and tissue replacement or modulation of host immune cells to create better conditions for healing.
- Stem cells may also be used in research applications such as toxicologic and pharmacologic screening, disease modeling, or studying developmental biology.
- Safety concerns associated with cell therapies generally relate to infectious agents, immunoreactions, and aberrant cell development.
- Multipotent mesenchymal stromal/stem cells have a higher safety profile compared with pluripotent stem cells.

INTRODUCTION

Stem cells are investigated for several reasons. In this article, the basic concepts and principles of stem cell biology as well as some key considerations for moving from bench to patient side are introduced. Excellent review articles are available in the veterinary literature on these topics to supplement this overview.[1–13]

EQUINE STEM CELL SOURCES

Definition of Stem Cells and Stromal Cells

Stem cells are defined as cells capable of self-renewal, proliferation, and differentiation. These properties should be demonstrated in vivo. In vivo, stemness can be

Department of Biomedical Sciences, Ontario Veterinary College, University of Guelph, 50 Stone Road East, Guelph, Ontario, N1G 2W1, Canada
* Corresponding author.
E-mail address: tkoch@uoguelph.ca

Vet Clin Equine 39 (2023) 461–474
https://doi.org/10.1016/j.cveq.2023.06.008

demonstrated by serial transplantation or germ-line transmission studies.[11] The concept of stem cell renewal is intriguing. The initial cell division of the stem cell is often referred to as "asymmetrical" cell division. It is a mitotic event, but intrinsic or extrinsic factors govern asymmetrical division of proteins and transcription factors within the cell. Thus, one of the initial daughter cells remains in the so-called stem cell niche to avoid depletion of the stem cell pool.[14,15] In contrast, the other daughter cell undergoes extensive proliferation and gives rise to a population of cells that eventually differentiates to the required cell type during cell replenishment. A hierarchical process of stem cell renewal, proliferation, and differentiation is apparent from this paradigm.

Current stem cell nomenclature is confusing and inconsistent in both human and veterinary medicine.[16] Various ways of categorizing and naming stem cells are discussed below.

Categories and Sources

Stem cells can be categorized based on their tissue of origin, their differentiation potential, or whether they are anchorage-dependent (adherent) or not.

Stem cell groups based on origin would include embryonic stem cells (ESCs), fetal and neonatal stem cells, and adult stem cells (**Fig. 1**). ESCs are, as the name implies, isolated from embryos. Fetal and neonatal cells are isolated from fetal samples or at the time of birth; umbilical cord tissue and cord blood are examples of neonatal cell sources. Adult stem cells are isolated from various tissues of the adult individual; examples include bone marrow and adipose tissue mesenchymal stromal cells (MSCs).

Sorting of stem cells based on their differentiation potential or cell potency would include the terms totipotent, pluripotent, multipotent, and unipotent cells. Totipotent cells can give rise to all the cells of the body as well as placental tissues; only the zygote is recognized as a totipotent cell. Pluripotent stem cells are capable of differentiating into all cell types of the body; embryonic and induced pluripotent stem cells belong to this group. Multipotent stem cells have a more limited differentiation potential but can give rise to several different cell types. Unipotent stem cells are typical resident tissue stem cells ensuring cell replenishment within specific tissues.

Adherent cells include embryonic, induced pluripotent, MSCs, and many progenitor cells, all of which require adherence to a substrate for expansion. Non-adherent stem cells do not attach to plastic culture dishes, cell feeder layers, or various extracellular matrices; CD34 positive hematopoietic stem cells that are used to treat human leukemia patients belong in this category but are stem cells nevertheless.[11] Equine hematopoietic stem cell research is at a nascent stage with few reports to date.[17]

Suspensions of nucleated cells from various tissues or solutions are sometimes referred to as stem cell preparations; these include the stromal vascular fraction (SVF) from adipose tissue and bone marrow aspirate concentrate (BMAC). MSCs or progenitor cells are present in SVF and BMAC, but unless the nucleated cell fraction is cultured for the propagation of these cells, they are present as only a tiny fraction of the cells provided.[18,19]

Pluripotent Stem Cells

ESCs are isolated from the inner cell mass of early-stage embryos (blastocysts). The cells adhere to fibroblast feeder cells initially but can later be expanded without feeder cells to provide a more homogenous cell population. These cells remain the gold standard for pluripotent cells and are capable of differentiating toward numerous cell fates in vitro and in vivo.[4,20]

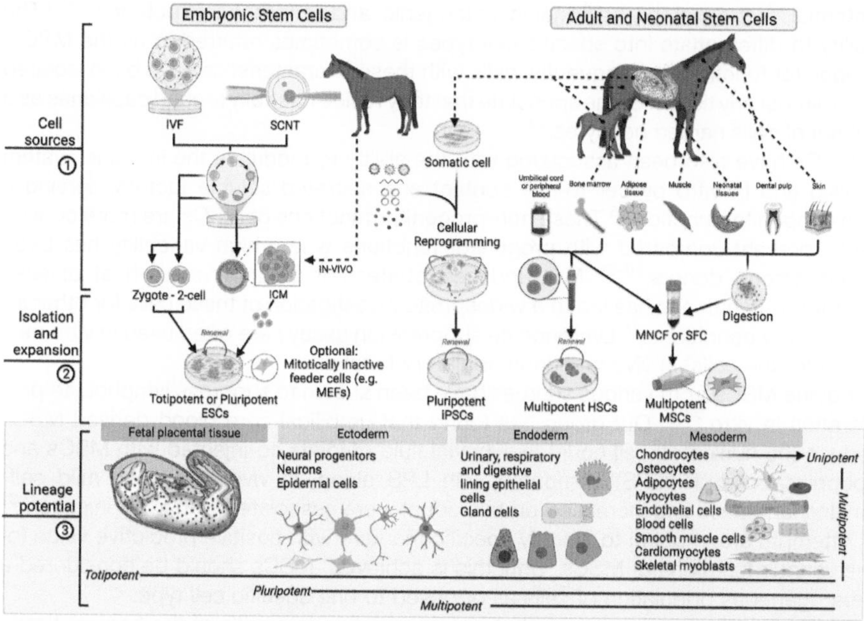

Fig. 1. Sources and differentiation capacity of equine stem cells. (1) and (2) Stem cells are characterized by their ability to self-renew (asymmetrical cell division), proliferate extensively in vitro, and differentiate into one or more tissue types. Stem cells can be derived from embryonic, fetal, neonatal, and adult tissues. Embryonic stem cells (ESCs) are most commonly isolated from the inner cell mass (ICM) of the blastocyst. Blastocysts can be produced in vivo after natural or artificial insemination or in vitro by somatic cell nuclear transfer (SCNT) or in vitro fertilization (IVF) techniques. Induced pluripotent stem cells (iPSCs) can be generated by reprogramming adult, neonatal, or fetal somatic cells to a pluripotent state using viral or nonviral transfection vectors and small molecule compounds. Mitotically arrested cellular feeder layers are often used for ESC and iPSC isolation and expansion, although human and mouse ESCs have been derived under feeder free conditions. Adult and neonatal stem cells are mononuclear cells and are isolated from the mononuclear cell fraction (MNCF). The MNCF from adipose tissue is often referred to as the stromal vascular fraction (SVF). (3) Totipotent cells can give rise to all cells of the body as well as placental tissues; only the zygote and blastomeres from two-cell embryos are recognized as a totipotent cell in equine development. Pluripotent stem cells can differentiate into cells from all three germ layers and form all cells of the body; ESCs and iPSCs belong to this group. Multipotent stem cells can give rise to cells from two germ layers or multiple cell types within one germ layer. If a stem cell can give rise to only one cell type, it is regarded as being unipotent.

Induced pluripotent stem cells (iPSCs) have circumvented the ethical issues surrounding ESCs and to some extent, the concerns of allogeneic use of ESCs. Inducing pluripotency refers to the process of reprogramming a differentiated somatic cell toward an ESC-like state using a few select transcription factors. Challenges to the iPSC technology includes the use of integrating viral vectors for transcription factor transduction, low efficiency of reprogramming, poor or partial reprogramming, and the realization that autologous use may be financially prohibitive.[21]

Mesenchymal Stromal Cells (Mesenchymal Stem Cells)

MSCs were initially isolated from bone marrow and characterized by adherence to polystyrene plastic cultureware, limited proliferation potential, and various differentiation potential in vitro, notably adipogenic, osteogenic, and chondrogenic potency.[22,23] The ability to differentiate into specific cell types is sometimes referred to as the MSC's progenitor function. Subsequently, cells with these characteristics have been isolated from almost any tissue. Some speculate that they reside naturally around capillaries as a subset of cells named pericytes.[24]

MSCs have also been associated with the ability to modulate the immune system in vivo and in vitro by cell-to-cell contact and secreted soluble factors, serving a non-progenitor function.[25] These non-progenitor functions of MSCs are more consistently present compared with progenitor functions where high variability has been noted among donors.[26–29] MSC-induced abatement of graft-versus-host disease symptoms in humans has led to a widespread investigation of these cells for other inflammatory conditions.[25] Lymphocyte suppression assays are often used in vitro as a proxy for the cells' in vivo immunomodulatory functions.

Equine MSCs from various sources have been shown to suppress lymphocyte proliferation in vitro.[26,30] Our group has found that umbilical cord blood-derived MSCs reduce the nucleated cell count in synovial fluid of joints co-injected with MSCs and lipopolysaccharide (LPS) compared with LPS alone, in vivo. However, mild self-limiting lameness and increased protein count were associated with MSC injection.[31]

Attempts are ongoing to identify specific markers with positive predictive value for the various functions of MSCs. Until this is achieved, MSCs should be considered a heterogeneous population of cells as opposed to one specific cell type.

Immature cells with a propensity for differentiation into cells of the harvest tissue and potentially other tissues have been isolated from several tissues including tendon, cartilage, synovial fluid, and dental pulp.[32–35]

EQUINE STEM CELL PRACTICES

Applications Overview

Stem cell applications can be broadly divided into four categories (**Fig. 2**).

1. Replacement strategies for failing cells and tissues
2. Immunomodulatory application of select stem cells, or stem cell-derived products, which exert regulatory effects on cells of the immune system
3. Toxicologic and pharmacologic screening of drug compounds
4. Developmental biology studies to gain insights into normal resident cell biology which may be used to design in situ regeneration strategies. The below is focused on the uses of above categories 1 and 2.

Administration Route and Hypodermic Needle Size

Direct intralesional injection has been the most common route of administration into tendons, tendon sheaths and synovial joints, but regional treatment using intra-arterial and intravenous (IV) administration is increasingly investigated and used.[36–38] Practical considerations such as whether hypodermic needle size affects the viability of injected cells have recently been investigated. Our group investigated various needle sizes and found that aspiration affects MSC viability, whereas injection does not.[39] Based on this, a large bore needle (18 ga or larger) is recommended for aspiration, but injection can be done using the most appropriate needle size for the circumstance.

Dose, Treatment Timing, and Frequency

There are currently no evidence-based recommendations as to the appropriate dose, treatment time, and frequency of treatment with MSCs or other cell products. Expert-based guidelines are moving toward delayed treatment (20–30 days post-injury),

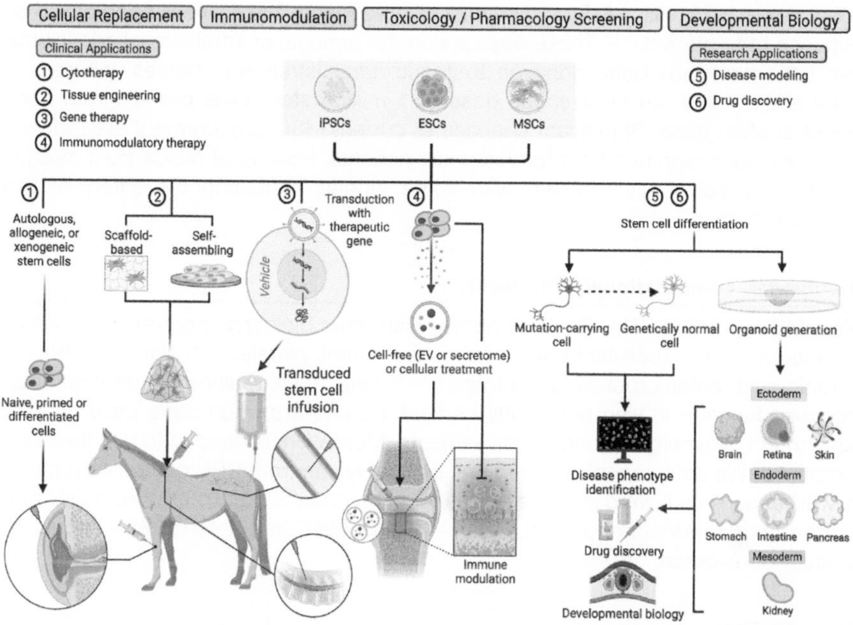

Fig. 2. Conceptual applications of equine stem cells. Stem cells can be used clinically by harnessing their progenitor functions for cellular replacement or non-progenitor functions for immunomodulation. Cellular replacement may involve (1) Cytotherapy or (2) tissue engineering where autologous, allogeneic, or xenogeneic stem cells are used to replace tissues or cells. (1) Cytotherapy is most commonly administered via direct intralesional injection into tendons or synovial fluid, but systemic and regional administrations are increasing. (2) Tissue engineering can occur by self-assembly or using a scaffold, which involves populating a synthetic or biologically derived matrix with stem cells and differentiating them into tissue-specific cells. The selection of a scaffold structure such as fibrous, microporous, monolithic, or hydrogel will depend on the desired tissue type. (3) Gene therapy involves treating patients with stem cells expressing a desired gene, allowing for targeted delivery of gene products such as vascular endothelial growth factor (VEGF) and basic fibroblast growth factor (FGF2) to assist recovery in specific regions. Cytotherapy, gene therapy, and tissue transplants are commonly combined with other biological compounds to facilitate effective delivery and maintain cell viability during injection. Immunomodulation involves using the (4) non-progenitor functions of stem cells such as their ability to regulate the immune system. Immunomodulatory treatments may involve administering soluble mediators (secretome), extracellular vesicles, or stem cells to sites of inflammation. In a research context, stem cells may be used for toxicology/pharmacology screening or studying developmental biology. (5) Disease modeling may be used to investigate developmental pathogenesis or test the efficacy and safety of drugs generally or patient specifically. (6) Disease modeling can be done by differentiating stem cells from patients with genetic conditions into afflicted cell types to gain insight into how pathogenic changes occur during development. Alternatively, stem cells can be genetically manipulated to correct mutations as a way of determining the importance of certain genes in pathogenesis or vice versa. Organoids are self-organizing; 3D cell cultures that are functionally and spatially characteristic of actual organs. Compared with 2D culture, organoids can more accurately model cell-to-cell interactions, organ development, and disease, which can also be used to better test drug efficacy and safety.

higher doses (>20 million MSCs), and multiple treatments 2 to 4 weeks apart based on response to treatment.[7,13] These dosages are for regional or intralesional administration. Little work has been done on systemic administration in horses, whereas in humans and mice, an intravenous dose of 1 million stem cells per kilogram body weight is often used. Significant changes to current MSC procurement are required to provide such high numbers for veterinary patients. Pooling of MSCs from multiple donors may solve this problem with some studies indicating the safety of this approach.[40–43]

Multimodal (Combinational) Treatments

Often MSCs, SVF, or BMAC are combined with other biological compounds such as autologous serum, acellular bone marrow supernatant, platelet-rich plasma (PRP), hyaluronic acid, antimicrobials, and others.[7,13,44] How these multimodal treatment approaches function in vivo are poorly understood and are often done based on the assumption of synergistic and additive effects. More work is needed to test these assumptions. We have recently shown that platelet lysate from PRP can be detrimental to MSC expansion in vitro in a dose-dependent manner.[45] Various antimicrobials may also be toxic to MSCs and combinational use of MSC and antimicrobial should be carefully considered.[44,46]

Transport Chain

SVF and BMAC can be procured in house and delivered within minutes to a few hours. Cultured cells can be delivered fresh within hours of detachment in hospitals with cell culture facilities. However, overnight transport of cells is commonly required. Both frozen and chilled cells are shipped at present.[13] How cell numbers, viability, and function are preserved through this transport chain is not fully understood.[47] We recently found that cryopreserved equine cord blood MSCs allowed to recover from cryogenic shock by culturing compared with immediately thawed MSCs equally suppressed lymphocytes proliferation in vitro.[48] The carrier solutions can also greatly influence cell recovery and viability. Increased focus is on using cell carrier products optimized for cell preservation, preferably excipients, which are cell carrier products that can be directly co-injected with the cells as opposed to ancillary carrier substances that have to be washed away from the cells before injection.[13]

Tissue Engineering

Stem cells have attracted significant interest for tissue engineering purposes due to their progenitor functions (see **Fig. 2**). Tissue engineering relies generally on a trio of factors including cells, scaffolds, and growth factors. Mechanical cues are increasingly considered for the generation of orthopedic tissues. Including mechanical stimulation, this quartet of factors for tissue engineering is referred to as the "diamond concept."[49]

Various scaffold printing technologies, such as three-dimensional (3D) bioprinting, are allowing for complex scaffold manufacturing applications as we have recently reviewed.[50] Bioprinting can be done based on patient images to provide patient-specific contoured implants. Synthetic or natural scaffold components can be combined with biological cues or enzymatic target sites. Scaffolds of different compositions and functionalization can be combined in 3D bioprints using the so-called "bioinks" in order best recapitulate biological tissues.

Gene Therapy

Gene therapy offers the potential for targeted gene expression of selected gene products (see **Fig. 2**). Advances are being made in gene therapy for the treatment of animals.[51] Combining gene therapy approaches with stem cell technologies may be of future use in horses.[52,53]

POTENTIAL SAFETY CONCERNS

Safety concerns associated with cell therapies generally relate to infectious agents, immunoreactions, and aberrant cell development (**Fig. 3**).[47] Unique safety concerns can be associated with the route of administration.

Infectious Agents

Infectious agents can be harbored within the cells and originate from the original donor animal of the cells or are introduced iatrogenically at any point from the environment during cell isolation and expansion, preparation of the cells for clinical use, at the time of treatment, or through contaminated products used in the manufacturing or administration of the cells. There are no tests developed specifically to screen initial source material for various infectious diseases in animals with no history or signs of disease.

A comprehensive layered biosecurity approach is therefore needed to reduce the risk of donor animal disease agents. Such considerations should include geography, travel history, medical history, farm management practices, physical and para-clinical monitoring of donor animals combined with diagnostic testing for infectious diseases considered a risk under the circumstances. Prior treatment with equine biologic products including antitoxins, plasma, and stem cells has also been associated with serum hepatitis.[54,55] Iatrogenic introduction of environmental infectious agents should be reduced through appropriate laboratory practices and product monitoring for infectious agents during the manufacturing process.

Culture media components, transport media of chilled cells, or cryomedia of frozen cell products may introduce infectious agents into the product.[47] Fetal bovine serum remains a critical component of equine cell culture despite its recognized drawbacks due to the absence of available serum-free or defined culture media for equine cells. Transmissible spongiform encephalopathies (TSEs) are a major concern of Fetal Bovine Serum (FBS) use, and there are no tests available to screen for the presence of TSE agents. A layered biosecurity approach is therefore deployed where FBS should be sourced from countries recognized as minimal risk.[56] Irradiation of FBS will further reduce the risk of bacterial and viral agents.[57]

Immunoreactions

Immunoreactions to a stem cell product could be due to the cells or adjuvant components within the product formulation or both. Stem cells are not immune-privileged as speculated by some in the past.[58] The cells do express Major Histocompatibility Complex Class I (MHC-I) to varying extent, and the cells are therefore recognized by the recipient immune system in cases of allogeneic or xenogeneic administration as demonstrated by the presence of antibody formation against the stem cells.[59] Interestingly, not all recipients develop an antibody response to non-tissue matched allogeneic cells, and, to date, no correlation between adverse reactions and antibody response has been reported. Haplotyping of cell preparations and haplotype matching between cells and recipient has been proposed as a way to reduce the risk of cell-induced adverse reactions and possibly increase dwell time of the cells within the recipient.[60] However, the single use of unmatched allogeneic cells seems safe with

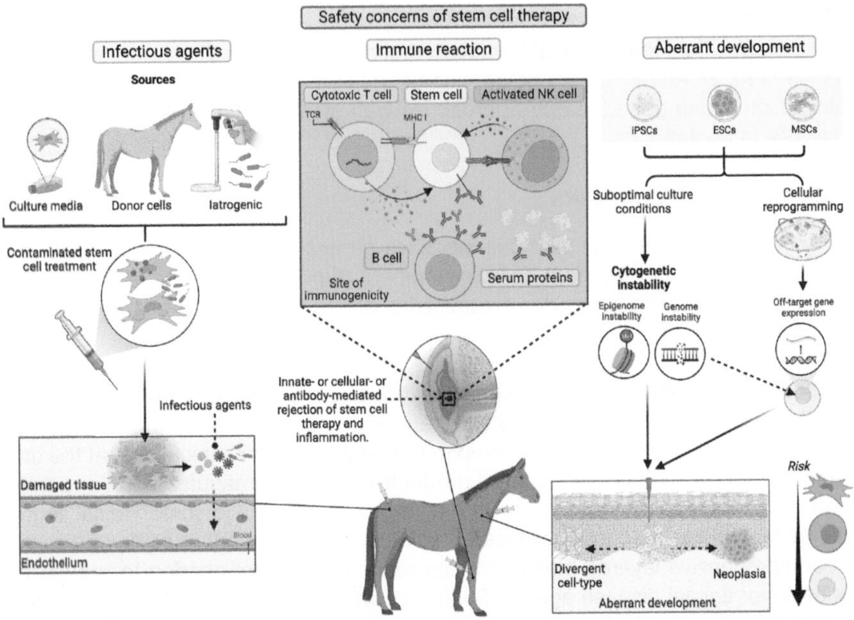

Fig. 3. Safety concerns of stem cell therapy. The main safety risks associated with stem cell therapy include contamination by infectious agents, immunogenicity, and aberrant cell development. Infectious agents may come from many different sources including donor cells, culture media, or the environment. Comprehensive biosecurity measures are necessary for mitigating the risk of treatment contamination. Immune reactions following cell therapy may result from the response of adaptive or innate immune components to foreign major histocompatibility complex class I (MHC-I) or antigens present on stem cells. Cell therapies may be rejected by cytotoxic CD8+ T-cell mediated cell-death, natural killer (NK) cells, components of the complement system, or neutralizing antibodies. Bovine serum proteins have also been shown to cause an immune reaction. Anti-inflammatory treatments consisting of frequent cold compress, bandaging, and non-steroidal anti-inflammatory drugs (NSAIDs) have been shown to be effective in mitigating immune reactions following administration of unmatched allogeneic cells. iPSCs may also be used for autologous treatments, mitigating the risk of immune rejection in recipients. Aberrant cell development refers to the spontaneous differentiation of stem cells to unwanted cell types. Cellular potency is a clinical risk given that pluripotent cells have the potential to become tumorigenic under certain conditions. Suboptimal laboratory conditions such as over-propagation, media choice, and oxygen tension may lead to cytogenetic instability in any cell-type, increasing the risk of tumorigenesis. Viral-mediated reprogramming of somatic cells to generate iPSCs poses unique risks that increase the chances of tumorigenesis, including a higher chance of chromosomal mutagenicity and the potential for off-target gene expression. Unlike most cells, iPSCs derived from karyotypically normal parental cells may show chromosomal aberrations in early passages, making cytogenetic screening and parental cell selection important considerations when using iPSCs for cytotherapy. However, iPSCs have a propensity to differentiate toward the lineage of their parental cell origin due to epigenetic memory, which could reduce the risk of aberrant development in clinical settings. Multipotent cell therapies present less of a risk considering that they are highly unlikely to form teratomas and their clinical utility is mainly related to non-progenitor functions such as cell–cell interactions and secretion of soluble factors.

common adverse reactions reported as self-limiting inflammatory responses of a few days duration that respond to standard anti-inflammatory treatments consisting of frequent cold compress, bandaging, and NSAIDs.[7,13] Although research into repeated administration of allogeneic equine MSCs is limited, studies show only mild or transient reaction to a second injection even in the absence of haplotype matching which has rarely been done in horses to date.[40,61–65] Further studies examining the effect of antibody response and in vivo cellular survival and efficacy are needed.

Bovine serum proteins have been proposed as a source of immune reactions.[64,66,67] We have recently reviewed attempts to reduce the presence of bovine proteins through rinsing of cells with FBS-free solutions before use and FBS replacement or reduction in the culture media hours or days before use have been explored.[68] The effect of such practices on reducing minor adverse reactions is not clear at the moment and should be weighed against possible reduced cell viability and functionality by serum depletion or reduction.

The final product may include several components to ensure cell viability during storage and transport and may be administered as part of a combinational product in conjunction with platelet lysate, PRP, acellular hematological suspensions such as bone marrow supernatant, hyaluronic acid, and dimethylsulfoxide (DMSO). These products may be associated with immune recognition and adverse reactions as well.

Although not an immunorecognition mechanism, thrombogenic events has been described with regional intravenous or intra-arterial cell infusion.[37] However, these complications were resolved if performed without the use of a tourniquet.[69] Since a tourniquet is required to obtain sufficient cell concentrations with regional IV administration, but is associated with thrombotic risks, the regional route of choice is now intra-arterial administration.

Aberrant Cellular Development

Aberrant cellular development where the cells spontaneously develop toward unwanted cell types has been proposed as a clinic risk due to pluripotent cells' ability to form teratomas in immunodeficient mice as proof of the cells' pluripotency. How the risk of teratoma formation in immunodeficient animals relates to clinical risk of neoplasia in immunocompetent animals is not well established.

Viral-based reprogramming methods for the creation of iPSCs or other cell enhancements may lead to genetic instability of the cells or unknown effects within the cells due to unintended off-target DNA changes within the cells.[21,70] This, in turn, could pose a risk if the cells are used clinically, justifying increased scrutiny of the cells the more engineered and manipulated they are. The risk of aberrant cell development seems very low, at present, when using multipotent stromal cells, because these cells can rarely form teratomas even in immunodeficient mice.[47]

Previously, it was hypothesized that undifferentiated multipotent MSCs would spontaneously differentiate into the desired cell fates at the injury site following direct injection into the damage tissue or organ, for example, tenocytes in tendons and chondrocytes in joints with cartilage damage. However, this theory has been debunked, and the beneficial effect of the cells is now hypothesized to be related to their non-progenitor functions through secreted factors and cell–cell contact with resident cells.[71,72] This observation, in turn, further lends evidence to the low risk of these cells unexpectedly becoming cells of concern in clinical cases. This said, multipotent mesenchymal stromal cells may become cytogenetically unstable as evidenced by abnormal karyotype due to extensive laboratory manipulation and cell expansion which in turn could increase the risk of these cells to become tumorigenic.[73] Karyotypic assessment is therefore recommended.

CLINICS CARE POINTS

- When contemplating clinical use of equine stem cells, the following should be considered:
- Are safety data available for the cells for the intended indication?
- Are efficacy data available for the cells for the intended indication?
- Is a certificate of analysis of the cells available for cell concentration, cell viability, sterility, and infectious disease testing?
- Has the context of the cell treatment been disclosed regarding experimental medicine or approved product and possible risks been discussed prior to obtaining informed owner consent?

DISCLOSURE

T. G. Koch is the founder and CEO of eQcell Inc.

FUNDING

T. G. Koch holds grant support from the Canadian Institutes of Health Research, Natural Sciences and Engineering Research Council of Canada, the Grayson Jockey Club and Equine Guelph. K. A. Russell is supported by a Mitacs Accelerate Award. A. G. Kuzma-Hunt is supported by scholarships from the Canadian Institutes of Health Research and the Ontario Veterinary College.

REFERENCES

1. De Schauwer C, Van de Walle GR, Van Soom A, et al. Mesenchymal stem cell therapy in horses: useful beyond orthopedic injuries? Vet Q 2013;33(4):234–41.
2. Fortier LA, Travis AJ. Stem cells in veterinary medicine. Stem Cell Res Ther 2011; 2(9):1–6.
3. de Bakker E, Van Ryssen B, De Schauwer C, et al. Canine mesenchymal stem cells: state of the art, perspectives as therapy for dogs and as a model for man. Vet Q 2013;33(4):225–33.
4. Hall V, Hinrichs K, Lazzari G, et al. Early embryonic development, assisted reproductive technologies, and pluripotent stem cell biology in domestic mammals. Vet J 2013;197(2):128–42.
5. Koh S, Piedrahita Ja. From "ES-like" cells to induced pluripotent stem cells: a historical perspective in domestic animals. Theriogenology 2014;81(1):103–11.
6. Lopez MJ, Jarazo J. State of the art: stem cells in equine regenerative medicine. Equine Vet J 2015;47(2):145–54.
7. Schnabel LV, Fortier LA, Wayne McIlwraith C, et al. Therapeutic use of stem cells in horses: which type, how, and when? Vet J 2013;197(3):570–7.
8. Volk SW, Theoret C. Translating stem cell therapies: the role of companion animals in regenerative medicine. Wound Repair Regen 2013;21(3):382–94.
9. Koch TG, Berg LC, Betts DH. Concepts for the clinical use of stem cells in equine medicine. Can Vet J 2008;49(10):1009–17.
10. Koch TG, Berg LC, Betts DH. Current and future regenerative medicine - principles, concepts, and therapeutic use of stem cell therapy and tissue engineering in equine medicine. The Canadian Veterinary Journal La Revue Veterinaire Canadienne 2009;50(2):155–65.

11. Voga M, Adamic N, Vengust M, et al. Stem Cells in Veterinary Medicine—Current State and Treatment Options. Front Vet Sci 2020;7. https://doi.org/10.3389/fvets.2020.00278.
12. Kamm JL, Riley CB, Parlane N, et al. Interactions between allogeneic mesenchymal stromal cells and the recipient immune system: a comparative review with relevance to equine outcomes. Front Vet Sci 2021;7. https://doi.org/10.3389/fvets.2020.617647.
13. Barrachina L, Romero A, Zaragoza P, et al. Practical considerations for clinical use of mesenchymal stem cells: from the laboratory to the horse. Vet J 2018; 238:49–57.
14. Berika M, Elgayyar ME, El-Hashash AHK. Asymmetric cell division of stem cells in the lung and other systems. Front Cell Dev Biol 2014;2. https://doi.org/10.3389/fcell.2014.00033.
15. Knoblich JA. Mechanisms of Asymmetric Stem Cell Division. Cell 2008;132(4): 583–97.
16. Viswanathan S, Shi Y, Galipeau J, et al. Mesenchymal stem versus stromal cells: International Society for Cell & Gene Therapy (ISCT®) Mesenchymal Stromal Cell committee position statement on nomenclature. Cytotherapy 2019;21(10): 1019–24.
17. Schwab UE, Tallmadge RL, Matychak MB, et al. Effects of autologous stromal cells and cytokines on differentiation of equine bone marrow–derived progenitor cells. AJVR (Am J Vet Res) 2017;78(10):1215–28.
18. Ruoss S, Walker JT, Nasamran CA, et al. Strategies to Identify Mesenchymal Stromal Cells in Minimally Manipulated Human Bone Marrow Aspirate Concentrate Lack Consensus. Am J Sports Med 2021;49(5):1313–22.
19. Bourin P, Bunnell BA, Casteilla L, et al. Stromal cells from the adipose tissue-derived stromal vascular fraction and culture expanded adipose tissue-derived stromal/stem cells: a joint statement of the International Federation for Adipose Therapeutics and Science (IFATS) and the International Society for Cellular Therapy (ISCT). Cytotherapy 2013;15(6):641–8.
20. Paterson Yz, Kafarnik C, Guest Dj. Characterization of companion animal pluripotent stem cells. Cytometry 2018;93(1):137–48.
21. Scarfone RA, Pena SM, Russell KA, et al. The use of induced pluripotent stem cells in domestic animals: a narrative review. BMC Vet Res 2020;16(1):477.
22. Friedenstein AJ, Chailakhyan RK, Gerasimov UV. Bone marrow osteogenic stem cells: in vitro cultivation and transplantation in diffusion chambers. Cell Tissue Kinet 1987;20(3):263–72.
23. Dominici M, Blanc KL, Mueller I, et al. Minimal criteria for defining multipotent mesenchymal stromal cells. The International Society for Cellular Therapy position statement. Cytotherapy 2006;8(4):315–7.
24. Caplan AI. All MSCs are pericytes? Cell Stem Cell 2008;3(3):229–30.
25. Tolar J, Le Blanc K, Keating A, et al. Concise review: hitting the right spot with mesenchymal stromal cells. Stem Cells (Dayton, Ohio) 2010;28(8):1446–55.
26. Tessier L, Bienzle D, Williams LB, et al. Phenotypic and immunomodulatory properties of equine cord blood-derived mesenchymal stromal cells. PLoS One 2015; 10(4). https://doi.org/10.1371/journal.pone.0122954.
27. Lee OJ. Steps towards standardized assessment and use of immunomodulatory mesenchymal stromal cells. Guelph, ON, Canada: University of Guelph; 2020.
28. Lepage SIM, Lee OJ, Koch TG. Equine cord blood mesenchymal stromal cells have greater differentiation and similar immunosuppressive potential to cord tissue mesenchymal stromal cells. Stem Cell Dev 2018;28(3):227–37.

29. Bagge J, Berg LC, Janes J, et al. Donor age effects on in vitro chondrogenic and osteogenic differentiation performance of equine bone marrow- and adipose tissue-derived mesenchymal stromal cells. BMC Vet Res 2022;18(1):388.
30. Carrade DD, Lame MW, Kent MS, et al. Comparative Analysis of the Immunomodulatory Properties of Equine Adult-Derived Mesenchymal Stem Cells. Cell Med 2012;4(1):1–12.
31. Williams LB, Koenig JB, Black B, et al. Equine allogeneic umbilical cord blood derived mesenchymal stromal cells reduce synovial fluid nucleated cell count and induce mild self-limiting inflammation when evaluated in an lipopolysaccharide induced synovitis model. Equine Vet J 2016;48(5):619–25.
32. Ishikawa S, Horinouchi C, Murata D, et al. Isolation and characterization of equine dental pulp stem cells derived from Thoroughbred wolf teeth. J Vet Med Sci 2017;79(1):47–51.
33. Murata D, Miyakoshi D, Hatazoe T, et al. Multipotency of equine mesenchymal stem cells derived from synovial fluid. Vet J 2014;202(1):53–61.
34. Lovati AB, Corradetti B, Lange Consiglio A, et al. Characterization and differentiation of equine tendon-derived progenitor cells. J Biol Regul Homeost Agents 2011;25(2 Suppl):S75–84.
35. Frisbie DD, McCarthy HE, Archer CW, et al. Evaluation of articular cartilage progenitor cells for the repair of articular defects in an equine model. J Bone Joint Surg 2015;97(6):484–93.
36. Knott LE, Fonseca-Martinez BA, O'Connor AM, et al. Current use of biologic therapies for musculoskeletal disease: A survey of board-certified equine specialists. Vet Surg 2022;51(4):557–67.
37. Sole A, Spriet M, Galuppo LD, et al. Scintigraphic evaluation of intra-arterial and intravenous regional limb perfusion of allogeneic bone marrow-derived mesenchymal stem cells in the normal equine distal limb using 99mTc-HMPAO. Equine Vet J 2012;44(5):594–9.
38. Espinosa P, Spriet M, Sole A, et al. Scintigraphic tracking of allogeneic mesenchymal stem cells in the distal limb after intra-arterial injection in standing horses. Vet Surg 2016;45(5):619–24.
39. Williams LB, Russell KA, Koenig JB, et al. Aspiration, but not injection, decreases cultured equine mesenchymal stromal cell viability. BMC Vet Res 2016;12(1):45.
40. Ardanaz N, Vázquez FJ, Romero A, et al. Inflammatory response to the administration of mesenchymal stem cells in an equine experimental model: effect of autologous, and single and repeat doses of pooled allogeneic cells in healthy joints. BMC Vet Res 2016;12(1):65.
41. Colbath AC, Dow SW, Hopkins LS, et al. Single and repeated intra-articular injections in the tarsocrural joint with allogeneic and autologous equine bone marrow-derived mesenchymal stem cells are safe, but did not reduce acute inflammation in an experimental interleukin-1β model of synovitis. Equine Vet J 2020;52(4):601–12.
42. Colbath AC, Dow SW, Hopkins LS, et al. Allogeneic vs. autologous intra-articular mesenchymal stem cell injection within normal horses: Clinical and cytological comparisons suggest safety. Equine Vet J 2020;52(1):144–51.
43. Williams LB, Co C, Koenig JB, et al. Response to intravenous allogeneic equine cord blood-derived mesenchymal stromal cells administered from chilled or frozen state in serum and protein-free media. Front Vet Sci 2016;3(56):1–13.
44. Russell KA, Garbin LC, Wong JM, et al. Mesenchymal stromal cells as potential antimicrobial for veterinary use—a comprehensive review. Front Microbiol 2020;11:606404.

45. Russell KA, Koch TG. Equine platelet lysate as an alternative to fetal bovine serum in equine mesenchymal stromal cell culture - too much of a good thing? Equine Vet J 2015;48(2):261–4.
46. Pezzanite L, Chow L, Soontararak S, et al. Amikacin induces rapid dose-dependent apoptotic cell death in equine chondrocytes and synovial cells in vitro. Equine Vet J 2020;52(5):715–24.
47. Devireddy LR, Boxer L, Myers MJ, et al. Questions and challenges in the development of mesenchymal stromal/stem cell-based therapies in veterinary medicine. Tissue Eng B Rev 2017;23(5):462–70.
48. Williams LB, Tessier L, Koenig JB, et al. Post-thaw non-cultured and post-thaw cultured equine cord blood mesenchymal stromal cells equally suppress lymphocyte proliferation in vitro. PLoS One 2014;9(12):e113615.
49. Giannoudis PV, Einhorn TA, Marsh D. Fracture healing: The diamond concept. Injury 2007;38(S4):S3–6.
50. Jamieson C, Keenan P, Kirkwood D, et al. A review of recent advances in 3D bioprinting with an eye on future regenerative therapies in veterinary medicine. Front Vet Sci 2021;7. https://doi.org/10.3389/fvets.2020.584193.
51. Thampi P, Samulski RJ, Grieger JC, et al. Gene therapy approaches for equine osteoarthritis. Front Vet Sci 2022;9. https://doi.org/10.3389/fvets.2022.962898.
52. Ball AN, Phillips JN, McIlwraith CW, et al. Genetic modification of scAAV-equine-BMP-2 transduced bone-marrow-derived mesenchymal stem cells before and after cryopreservation: An "off-the-shelf" option for fracture repair. J Orthop Res 2019;37(6):1310–7.
53. Reisbig NA, Pinnell E, Scheuerman L, et al. Synovium extra cellular matrices seeded with transduced mesenchymal stem cells stimulate chondrocyte maturation in vitro and cartilage healing in clinically-induced rat-knee lesions in vivo. PLoS One 2019;14(3):e0212664.
54. Divers TJ, Tomlinson JE, Tennant BC. The history of Theiler's disease and the search for its aetiology. Vet J 2022;287:105878.
55. Tomlinson JE, Kapoor A, Kumar A, et al. Viral testing of 18 consecutive cases of equine serum hepatitis: A prospective study (2014-2018). J Vet Intern Med 2019; 33(1):251–7.
56. European Commission. Note for guidance on minimising the risk of transmitting animal spongiform encephalopathy agents via human and veterinary medicinal products (EMA/410/01 rev.3). 2011.
57. Committee for Medicinal Products for Human Use. Guideline on the use of bovine serum in the manufacture of human biological medicinal products (EMA/CHMP/BWP/457920/2012 rev 1). 2013.
58. Ankrum Ja, Ong JF, Karp JM. Mesenchymal stem cells: immune evasive, not immune privileged. Nat Biotechnol 2014;32(3):252–60.
59. Berglund AK, Fortier LA, Antczak DF, et al. Immunoprivileged no more: measuring the immunogenicity of allogeneic adult mesenchymal stem cells. Stem Cell Res Ther 2017;8(1):1–7.
60. Rowland AL, Miller D, Berglund A, et al. Cross-matching of allogeneic mesenchymal stromal cells eliminates recipient immune targeting. STEM CELLS Translational Medicine 2020;10(5):694–710.
61. Van Hecke L, Magri C, Duchateau L, et al. Repeated intra-articular administration of equine allogeneic peripheral blood-derived mesenchymal stem cells does not induce a cellular and humoral immune response in horses. Vet Immunol Immunopathol 2021;239:110306.

62. Depuydt E, Broeckx SY, Chiers K, et al. Cellular and Humoral Immunogenicity Investigation of Single and Repeated Allogeneic Tenogenic Primed Mesenchymal Stem Cell Treatments in Horses Suffering From Tendon Injuries. Front Vet Sci 2022;8. https://doi.org/10.3389/fvets.2021.789293.
63. Magri C, Schramme M, Febre M, et al. Comparison of efficacy and safety of single versus repeated intra-articular injection of allogeneic neonatal mesenchymal stem cells for treatment of osteoarthritis of the metacarpophalangeal/metatarsophalangeal joint in horses: A clinical pilot study. PLoS One 2019;14(8):e0221317.
64. Joswig A-J, Mitchell A, Cummings KJ, et al. Repeated intra-articular injection of allogeneic mesenchymal stem cells causes an adverse response compared to autologous cells in the equine model. Stem Cell Res Ther 2017;8(1):42.
65. Muñoz AM. Evaluation of repeated intralesional injection of allogeneic umbilical equine cord blood mesenchymal stromal cells for treatment of equine Superficial digital flexor tendonitis. Guelph, ON, Canada: University of Guelph; 2023.
66. Rowland AL, Burns ME, Levine GJ, et al. Preparation Technique Affects Recipient Immune Targeting of Autologous Mesenchymal Stem Cells. Front Vet Sci 2021;8: 1050.
67. Longhini ALF, Salazar TE, Vieira C, et al. Peripheral blood-derived mesenchymal stem cells demonstrate immunomodulatory potential for therapeutic use in horses. PLoS One 2019;14(3):e0212642.
68. Pilgrim CR, McCahill KA, Rops JG, et al. A review of fetal bovine serum in the culture of mesenchymal stromal cells and potential alternatives for veterinary medicine. Front Vet Sci 2022;9. https://doi.org/10.3389/fvets.2022.859025.
69. Trela JM, Spriet M, Padgett KA, et al. Scintigraphic comparison of intra-arterial injection and distal intravenous regional limb perfusion for administration of mesenchymal stem cells to the equine foot. Equine Vet J 2014;46(4):479–83.
70. Arzi B, Webb TL, Koch TG, et al. Cell Therapy in Veterinary Medicine as a Proof-of-Concept for Human Therapies: Perspectives From the North American Veterinary Regenerative Medicine Association. Front Vet Sci 2021;8.
71. Sipp D, Robey PG, Turner L. Clear up this stem-cell mess. Nature 2018; 561(7724):455–7.
72. Caplan AI. Mesenchymal Stem Cells: Time to Change the Name. Stem Cells Translational Medicine 2017;6(6):1445–51.
73. Alizadeh AH, Briah R, Villagomez DAF, et al. Cell identity, proliferation, and cytogenetic assessment of equine umbilical cord blood mesenchymal stromal cells. Stem Cell Dev 2018;27(24):1729–38.

Use of Stem Cells for the Treatment of Musculoskeletal Injuries in Horses

Ashlee E. Watts, DVM, PhD, DACVS*

KEYWORDS

• Mesenchymal stem cell • Mesenchymal stromal cell • Musculoskeletal • MSC • Horse • Orthopedic

KEY POINTS

- There are no Food and Drug Administration–approved equine MSC therapies in the United States.
- There is good evidence with rigorous and objective end points of a beneficial effect of MSC therapy for injury to the superficial digital flexor tendon.
- There is good evidence that MSCs are generally safe.
- Adverse immune reaction to MSC therapy is likely when allogeneic (non-self-derived) or laboratory-contaminated MSCs are used, especially if the therapy is used more than once.
- The primary concern of adverse immune reaction is not the clinically recognizable adverse response but the destruction of MSCs because dead MSCs are nonfunctional MSCs.

INTRODUCTION

Whether a backyard pony, a weekend horse show warrior, or an international competition horse, horses are intended to be athletic by their owners. Athleticism requires a healthy and sound musculoskeletal system, which is compromised by wear-and-tear injuries, accidental injuries, and developmental abnormalities. Although a slew of symptom-modifying treatments are available to the veterinarian to treat musculoskeletal problems, a disease-modifying treatment is not available. It should be no surprise that equine veterinarians and horse owners alike have an intense interest in regenerative therapies that could be disease modifying and improve long-term outcomes over currently available therapies.

Mesenchymal stem, or stromal, cells (MSCs) have been used as a regenerative therapy in horses for musculoskeletal injury since the late 1990s and in some regions have become standard of care for certain injuries.[1–3] Yet, there is no Food and Drug

10310 Dyess Road, College Station, TX 77845, USA
* Corresponding author.
E-mail address: ashleewattsdvm@gmail.com

Vet Clin Equine 39 (2023) 475–487
https://doi.org/10.1016/j.cveq.2023.07.003
vetequine.theclinics.com

Administration–approved MSC therapeutic in the United States for horses. In humans, lack of regulatory approval in the United States has been caused by failure of late-phase clinical trials to demonstrate consistent therapeutic effects.[4–6] Nonuniformity of MSC preparation and application techniques contribute to this lack of consistent effects.[5,7,8]

Like the human field, the selection, preparation, and application of equine MSCs is wildly nonuniform in every way possible: tissue source, autologous versus allogeneic, preparation technique, and application technique. The most used equine MSC products in musculoskeletal applications include the minimally manipulated products, adipose-derived stromal fraction and bone marrow aspirate concentrate, or the culture expanded products, adipose-derived MSC and bone marrow-derived MSC, whereas MSCs from peripheral blood and umbilical cord or blood have received limited attention. Autologous (donor and recipient are the same horse) and allogeneic (the donor and recipient are different horses) products have been used. Fresh and frozen products have been used. Culture medium, blood products, and bone marrow products have been used as a vehicle for injection. Finally, laboratory processes to culture MSCs or even to define MSCs are different from every laboratory. Unfortunately, there are more differences than there are similarities between the reported equine MSC products, making comparisons between them and deciphering the best possible treatment nearly impossible. However, among all the confusion, MSCs continue to hold great promise and their investigation remains worth the effort.

Regarding the types of musculoskeletal injury that MSCs have been used to treat, the differences continue. Equine MSCs have been applied to acute and chronic injury, tendon and ligament injury, cartilage injury and osteoarthritis, and bone lesions.

It is entirely possible that among all these different MSC products and MSC preparation techniques there is an ideal "one" for each category of musculoskeletal injury. As such, considerable efforts have been made to prime or precondition MSCs for specific diseases.[9,10] However, it is also possible that the ideal MSC therapeutic would have benefit for all musculoskeletal injuries, acute and chronic. Although this "cures what ails you" approach sounds a bit questionable, given the natural state of the MSC, to assist in tissue maintenance and repair, and to be exquisitely responsive to the local environment, it can be defended. In one study, equine MSCs from different tissue sources were heterogenous in their baseline expression of immune-related genes, which is well known; however, following interferon-γ stimulation MSC gene expression responded similarly, confirming that different preparations of MSCs are likely to respond similarly in an inflamed environment in vivo.[11] Arnold Caplan's moniker for the MSC, the "medicinal signaling cell," supports the notion that a single MSC product could be useful in diverse disease applications.[12,13]

DISCUSSION

Mesenchymal Stem Cells for Tendon and Ligament

Injury of the superficial digital flexor tendon (SDFT) constitutes approximately half of all racehorse injuries, affects one-quarter of racehorses in training, and is commonly injured in sport horses.[14,15] These overstrain injuries occur when exercise-induced degenerative changes accumulate over time, eventually resulting in fibrillar slippage and breakage of cross-linking with resultant tendon rupture and tendon tearing.[16] Although tendons heal well they do not regenerate, and instead heal with inferior scar tissue.[17,18] This hypercellular scar tissue has reduced elasticity and is biomechanically inferior, which contributes to poor functional recovery and a high risk of reinjury.[19] The frequency of injury and unacceptable outcomes is likely why MSC use in horses was first reported in tendon and ligament and also why tendon has been the most frequently reported structure to be treated with MSCs in the horse.[20]

The first clinical description of MSC use in horses was in 2001 in the form of raw bone marrow to the suspensory ligament by Herthel.[21] Two years later Roger Smith's group published a case report of a pony treated and then in 2008 more than 500 horses treated with culture-expanded autologous bone marrow–derived MSCs by intralesional injection to the injured SDFT.[22,23] The same group published the first large study of culture-expanded MSCs that showed improved outcomes of MSC-treated tendons 11 years later in 2012. It was a retrospective report on the treatment of 141 client-owned racehorses treated with autologous bone marrow–derived MSCs suspended in bone marrow supernatant by intralesional injection. Horses were followed up for at least 2 years after return to full work. The reinjury rate of 25% for National Hunt (n = 105) racehorses was significantly better than previous publications.[18] This was an exciting paper that sparked substantial interest in MSC use for tendon injury; however, it was plagued with the criticism that is typical for retrospectives studies (there were no control treatments, no blinding, or random allocation).

To address the lack of control subjects, blinding, and random allocation, the same group collected 12 horses with career-ending naturally occurring SDFT injury. The horses were randomly assigned to treatment with 10 million autologous bone marrow–derived MSCs suspended in 2 mL of marrow supernatant or the same volume of saline. Following a 6-month controlled exercise program the horses were euthanized and tendons were assessed. MSC-treated tendons were substantially improved compared with control animals; they had lower structural stiffness, lower histologic scoring of organization and crimp pattern, lower cellularity, lower DNA content, less vascularity, lower water content, lower glycosamionglycan (GAG) content, and reduced matrix metalloproteinase-13 activity.[2] This study provided prospective, blinded evidence of superiority of MSC therapy to controlled exercise alone but had some limitations. First, the control injection of saline would be expected to be proinflammatory immediately following injection and could have worsened the outcome in the control group. Using the MSC injection vehicle of bone marrow supernatant as the control injection would have been an interesting comparison. Second, although the horses entered the trial with naturally occurring injury, they did not complete a full controlled exercise program with return to race training and competition. It is possible that the marked improvements in multiple parameters at 6 months following treatment would not have translated to improved tendon durability. This certainly was the case in an equine experimental model of resurfacing cartilage injury with MSCs where early improvement because of MSC therapy were not maintained longer-term.[24]

The first clinical report of allogeneic MSCs for tendon was another retrospective study. Fifty-two warmblood horses with injury of the SDFT, suspensory ligament, deep digital flexor tendon, or inferior check ligament from two different equine hospitals were treated with cultured umbilical cord blood–derived MSCs. About 2 to 10 million cells per lesion were administered and some lesions were treated twice. The owners reported a return to full work at the same or higher level in 40 (77%) of horses. Neither the structure nor the age of the horse affected the outcome.[25] The major criticism of this report is the primary use of retrospective, owner-reported outcomes and the lack of a comparison group, either concurrent or historical.

A recent retrospective report compared outcomes after autologous bone marrow–derived MSCs and allogeneic adipose-derived MSCs for the treatment of SDFT injury in racehorses. Although retrospective, this study is remarkable because it includes a large number of horses, has a contemporaneous control group, and long-term follow-up that is objective and rigorous. A total of 213 Thoroughbred racehorses with SDFT injury were included, all of which received the same 12-month controlled exercise program; 66 also received intralesional autologous bone marrow–derived MSC and 17 received allogeneic adipose-derived MSC treatment. Follow-up was a minimum of 2 years after return to full race training. Compared with controlled exercise alone, autologous MSC treatment was associated with increased odds of returning to racing (odds ratio, 3.19; 95% confidence interval, 1.55–6.81) and increased odds of completing at least five races postinjury (odds ratio, 2.64; 95% confidence interval, 1.32–5.33), whereas there were no improvements associated with treatment with allogeneic MSCs.[1] Although this study was retrospective, it is reasonable evidence that intralesional treatment with autologous bone marrow–derived MSCs is associated with long-term improvements in tendon healing. Unfortunately, it is not possible to know why the adipose-derived MSCs did not result in improvements. It could have been because they were allogeneic, and the resultant immune response rendered the cells ineffective. It could have been inherent differences in MSCs from adipose versus bone marrow. It could have been the timing of treatment because there was an inevitable treatment delay for autologous MSCs as compared with allogeneic, which were available nearly immediately on diagnosis. Finally, it could have been the cell dose, because it was only 10 million for the bone marrow MSCs and 21 million for the adipose MSCs; however, lower doses have been implicated in reduced effect previously.[26]

Although no large, placebo-controlled and randomized clinical trials are available, there is good evidence in the literature that autologous MSCs improve tendon repair in the horse. Unfortunately, it remains unknown whether MSCs are doing this by differentiating into tendon cells and regenerating tendon tissue or by modulating the inflammation and the resultant repair process or both. For either mechanism, it seems logical that the time of optimal time of treatment following tendon or ligament injury would be before accumulation of fibrous scar tissue and/or before peak inflammation; however, this is not yet known.[1] If early treatment is important to the mechanism of repair, allogeneic MSCs would allow earlier treatment, avoiding the time to isolate and expand autologous MSCs. However, the best evidence in naturally occurring SDFT injury is supportive of improved outcomes when autologous bone marrow–derived MSCs are used, suggesting that this 3- to 4-week delay is not a detriment to MSC therapy.[1]

Mesenchymal Stem Cells for Osteoarthritis

Cartilage injury and osteoarthritis are a common cause of lameness in horses for which there are no approved disease-modifying treatments.[27] In vitro studies have demonstrated that MSCs produce cartilage-specific substances that could improve cartilage repair, such as aggrecan, glycosaminoglycans, and collagen type II.[9,28,29] Experimental studies for cartilage resurfacing indicate improvements in acute cartilage injury and intra-articular fracture.[24,30,31] Despite the early evidence of benefits for acute cartilage injury and osteoarthritis and European Medicines Agency (EMA) marketing approval, there have only been a few clinical publications on MSC use in the horse.

The first clinical report in the literature for intra-articular use of MSCs in horses was in 2009. Autologous bone marrow–derived MSCs were administered by intra-articular injection to the stifles of 33 horses that had received arthroscopic surgery for stifle injury after lameness was localized to the stifle by diagnostic anesthesia. At an average follow-up of 24 months, 43% of horses returned to their previous level of work, 33% returned to work, and 24% failed to return to work. In the 24 horses diagnosed with meniscal injury, 75% returned to work compared with 60% in historical reports that did not receive MSCs following arthroscopy.[32] The retrospective nature, owner-reported outcomes, and the lack of control subjects other than historical reports are the main criticisms of this study.

In a prospective and controlled study, autologous adipose-derived MSCs were used in horses with lameness because of distal tarsal osteoarthritis. Horses were treated with intra-articular injections of autologous stem cells (treated), intra-articular injection with corticosteroid (control), and untreated (no treatment control). There were long-term beneficial effects of MSCs when compared with corticosteroid, which had greater short-term improvements.[33]

A more recent field study was performed seeking regulatory approval by the EMA for the use of allogeneic adipose-derived MSCs in horses with osteoarthritis. Thirty-seven horses were treated with adipose-derived allogeneic MSCs by intra-articular injection, whereas 33 horses received a control treatment. At 90 days follow-up, MSC-treated horses had improved lameness compared with control animals, but marketing authorization was not granted because of safety concerns among other concerns.[34,35]

Another recent report compared one or two intra-articular injections of allogeneic umbilical cord–derived MSCs to the fetlock for the treatment of lameness because of osteoarthritis. Twenty-eight horses were divided into two groups for two blinded treatment injections, 1 month apart. Group 1 received an MSC injection and a placebo injection 1 month later. Group 2 received MSC at both injection time points. All horses underwent an 8-week controlled exercise program. Lameness improved over the 6-month duration of the study after treatment but there was no benefit of the second intra-articular injection.[36] The lack of beneficial effect of the second allogeneic injection could be caused by immune recognition with subsequent destruction of MSCs because they were not major histocompatibility complex (MHC)-matched between the donor and the recipient.[37] A similar study using an autologous MSC would be interesting.

There are two currently approved MSC therapeutics by the EMA. One approved product, HorStem, is an allogeneic umbilical cord–derived MSCs product for the treatment of osteoarthritis. Work on this product demonstrating efficacy as lameness reduction 60 days after treatment and safety up to 2 years was not published in peer reviewed literature but was part of a graduate dissertation. It was randomized, blinded, placebo controlled, and multicenter. Horses were eligible if they had lameness that was localized to a joint with mild to moderate radiographically apparent osteoarthritis. The primary outcome was lameness improvement at 60 days following treatment injection. There are a few limitations of this study. The distribution of joints was not homogenous with more pastern joints in the placebo group. The athletic purpose of enrolled horses was heterogenous; most were used for "leisure" (38%) and equestrian lessons (24%), and the remaining had more rigorous expectations of jumping (19%) and dressage (19%). Saline was the placebo injection, which would be expected to induce mild posttreatment inflammation.[38]

The other EMA-approved MSC product, Arti-Cell FORTE, is also allogeneic but is chondrogenic-induced peripheral blood–derived MSCs. There are a few clinical reports of these cells for joint disease. The first was a preliminary study of 20 horse fetlocks, split into four groups: (1) platelet-rich plasma (PRP), (2) MSCs, (3) MSCs + PRP, or (4) chondrogenic-induced MSCs + PRP.[28] The second was a pilot study with 165 horses, using multiple joints including coffin (43), pastern (34), fetlock (58), and stifle (30) treated with either MSCs + PRP (n = 49) or chondrogenic-induced MSCs + PRP (n = 116).[39] In a final study, 50 horses with mild fetlock joint disease received intra-articular injection of 2 million chondrogenic-induced MSCs suspended in plasma, and 25 horses were injected with saline. Following injection up to 18 weeks there was improved lameness, effusion, and joint flexion response in MSC-treated horses. After 1 year, more MSC-treated horses were in work compared with the saline-treated.[40] Similar to other studies, saline was used as the control and transient inflammation would be expected following saline injection to the joint. An interesting comparison would have been the same allogeneic plasma used as the control injection, rather than saline. In a previous study, this group also documented lack of humoral immune response to their MSCs, which they attributed to transforming growth factor-β treatment of MSCs. Unfortunately, blood collection for antibody assays was performed once, between 5 and 553 days after MSC injection, which is not an adequate protocol for detection of humoral response.[41] It would be interesting to repeat this study with more stringent analysis of humoral immune response, because lack of rigor has also led to false assessment of antibody production in human MSC trials.[42,43]

Mesenchymal Stem Cells for Bone

Despite numerous publications on MSCs for the treatment of bone pathologies in humans, there has been little published on MSCs for the treatment of bone pathologies in the horse.[44]

In a retrospective report the results for treatment of subchondral bone cysts in the stifles of unraced Thoroughbreds with surgical debridement, intralesional bone marrow–derived autologous MSCs, or intralesional corticosteroid were compared. There were no differences in the proportion of horses that were able to race posttreatment: 41/57 (72%) of horses treated by arthroscopic debridement raced, 16/19 (84%) of horses treated with intralesional MSCs raced, and 21/31 (68%) of horses treated with intralesional corticosteroids raced.[45] This retrospective study suggests that autologous MSCs have similar outcomes to other well-accepted modes of treatment. An interesting study would be a prospective and randomized application of the three different treatments.

Challenges for Clinical Mesenchymal Stem Cell Use for Musculoskeletal Applications

There is still insufficient evidence of MSC effectiveness in horses. This is not surprising, because even in humans, prospective randomized phase III trials have yet to provide clear evidence of MSC efficacy for musculoskeletal applications. This apparent failure of MSCs may be secondary to the incomplete understanding, which has not allowed optimization of MSC therapy. There are several challenges that need to be better understood to optimize musculoskeletal MSC therapy and facilitate marketing approval.

- Without a clear in vivo mechanism of action, it is not possible to design appropriate potency assays or relevant clinical end points.
- Whether the in vitro differences in MSC phenotype and function that differ based on tissue source, donor age, or culture techniques predict their effectiveness in the patient remains unknown.
- Although acute rejection responses generally do not occur, and local reactions are mild and transient, there is a negative effect of the immune response to allogeneic MSCs on efficacy.
- Repeated use of noncrossmatched MSCs should be avoided, because a humoral immune response against the injected MSCs would be expected.
- Although IgG responses against laboratory contaminants to MSCs cause increased inflammation and immune destruction of contaminated MSCs, even more alarming is the possibility of an IgE response to bovine contaminants.

- A dead MSC is a nonfunctional MSC, so although there may be no long-term negative consequence of MSC therapy that is recognized as foreign by the immune system, there would be no benefit.

The mechanisms of MSC therapy remain unknown: is it tissue replacement, modulation of tissue repair, modulation of immune function, or something else? There are numerous in vitro studies that document anabolic, chemotactic, inflammatory, anti-inflammatory, and immune-mediated activity of MSCs. Demonstrating the mechanism of MSC function in vivo is much more difficult. Without a clear in vivo mechanism of action, it is not possible to design appropriate potency assays or relevant clinical end points. One study demonstrated that MSCs enhanced endogenous progenitor recruitment to injected joints in the horse.[37] This mechanism would be particularly useful for the aged equine patient, because the endogenous progenitor concentration within synovial fluid declines with age and is likely responsible for age-related progression of osteoarthritis.[46,47]

Although MSCs from all sources share similarities, including self-renewal ability, multipotency, and immunomodulation abilities, heterogeneity of MSCs prevails. Whether the in vitro differences in MSC phenotype and function that differ based on tissue source, culture techniques, or donor variability predict their effectiveness in the patient remains unknown. There has been much published about the heterogeneity between different tissue sources of MSCs and different claims have been made as to the ideal tissue source for each application of MSCs. However, when tissue sources were sampled multiple times from the same donor, there was similar heterogeneity, suggesting this could be an in vitro phenomenon.[48] Further support that in vitro MSC phenotype might not predict function is that the variability in inflammation-related gene expression from different tissue sources became more similar after interferon-γ stimulation, suggesting that MSC will respond similarly to each other in an inflammatory environment when used clinically.[11] Finally, the characteristics of the patient and of the disease state during MSC therapy are likely to affect MSC function, introducing another source of variability in MSC function.

A concern that impacts allogeneic MSC use is that MSCs are no longer considered to be immune-privileged and donor-specific antibody production against allogeneic MSCs has been confirmed in people[4,49,50] and horses.[37,51–55] Although acute rejection responses generally do not occur, and local reactions are mild and transient, there is a negative effect of the immune response to allogeneic MSCs on efficacy.[37] In the horse, endogenous progenitor recruitment was enhanced after autologous and MHC-matched allogeneic MSC injection but not after MHC mismatched allogeneic injection.[37] This is an important mechanistic finding because synovial MSCs are likely responsible for articular cartilage repair in the native joint, and their reduced concentration during aging is in part responsible for age-related osteoarthritis.[46,47]

Yet, the MSC is still immune evasive, and able to persist longer and induce markedly less inflammation than a non-MSC mismatched cell transplant.[56] Certainly, there is evidence of allogeneic MSC tolerance in the horse without overt rejection responses after allogeneic MSC therapy and two equine allogeneic MSC products have a marketing authorization by the EMA.[3] However, repeated treatments of MSCs from a donor with the same MHC haplotype would be expected to suffer immune rejection and MSC destruction. This has been demonstrated in preclinical models, where syngeneic (donor and recipient are genetically similar and immunologically compatible) and noncrossmatched allogeneic MSC improved outcomes after the first use, but only syngeneic MSCs were effective on additional treatments. Therefore, repeated use of noncrossmatched MSCs should be avoided, because a humoral immune response against the injected MSCs would be expected.[57]

It should be kept in mind, that even at the first administration, there can be a humoral immune response against the allogeneic MSCs. This is because antibodies against the donor MHC can exist, despite lack of previous MSC exposure. This presensitization is known to occur after blood transfusion and pregnancy; however, anti-MHC antibodies can develop because of cross reactivity with epitopes on other antigens.[42,58,59]

A final consideration is the effect the laboratory culture period can have on MSC safety and even MSC effectiveness. It has been shown that bovine protein contaminants from the culture medium used to nourish MSCs can cause marked inflammation and antibody-induced cytotoxicity of injected MSCs.[55,60] Although it had been reported that bovine contamination of MSCs is not clinically relevant in cats and horses because of lack of change in titers against bovine[61,62] it is more likely that antibovine titers are simply too high to allow for amnestic responses after further bovine exposure.[60] Although these IgG responses would cause increased inflammation and immune destruction of contaminated MSCs, even more alarming is the possibility of an IgE response to bovine contaminants.[63]

Local adverse response, or joint flare, is known to occur in 10% to 20% of horses following intra-articular MSC administration and is secondary to immune recognition of a foreign substance.[32,38] The increased incidence of immune reaction after musculoskeletal use of MSCs as opposed to other applications is because MSCs are typically injected locally for musculoskeletal therapy, within a tendon core lesion or by intra-articular injection. For the synovial joint, the large volume to small surface area ratio and a blood-joint barrier limits diffusion of small molecules and transport of proteins.[64,65] For tendon, hypovascularity and dense matrix maintain MSCs at the site of injection.[66] These unique characteristics have allowed documentation of clinically recognizable adverse responses to mismatched allogeneic MSCs and fetal bovine serum contaminated MSCs.[37,60] However, the focus should not be on the adverse response, which is mild, likely because of the profound immune-modulating effects of MSCs. Rather, the focus should be on the cytotoxicity against MSCs that results from these immune responses. A dead MSC is a nonfunctional MSC, so although there may be no long-term negative consequence of MSC therapy, there would be no benefit.[57]

SUMMARY

Commercial interests have had a strong influence on the discussion of the advantages of allogeneic over autologous MSCs, different tissue sources, different donor ages, and different culture techniques rather than the biologic merits that affect efficacy and safety. Certainly, there are several distinct commercial advantages for allogeneic MSC therapy.[67] Despite these proprietary advantages, it is intriguing that most human tendon injury clinical trials[68] and osteoarthritis clinical trials[69] use autologous MSCs. This is not the case for intra-articular use in the horse, where most reports use allogeneic therapy, but it is true for reports on clinical equine tendon injury where autologous use has prevailed. A recent retrospective study compared the outcomes after autologous and allogeneic MSC therapy in racehorses with tendon injury. They found significant improvements in racing outcomes after autologous therapy, but not allogeneic.[1] In bone, the only equine clinical report used autologous MSCs.[45]

Despite the lack of Food and Drug Administration approval of an MSC therapeutic in the United States, there is good evidence that the treatment is safe and effective in the horse. It is hoped that, with continued work and careful design of clinical trials, an MSC therapeutic will meet the promise that has been held for so many years and equine veterinarians will have an effective and safe commercially available therapeutic to improve musculoskeletal injury outcomes in horses.

CLINICS CARE POINTS

- There are no FDA-approved equine MSC therapeutics in the United States.
- Adverse reactions to MSC therapy can occur because of laboratory contamination of MSCs or because of immune rejection of allogeneic MSCs.
- The primary concern of adverse immune reaction to MSCs is not the clinically recognizable adverse response, which is mild and nearly undetectable in most cases, but the destruction of MSCs because dead MSCs are nonfunctional MSCs.
- Donor selection and MSC preparation technique can reduce immune recognition of allogeneic MSCs, but cannot overcome it, unless the donor and recipient are immune compatible.
- Repeated treatments of allogeneic MSCs should be avoided because a humoral immune response would be expected after a second exposure.
- When immune monitoring is performed after allogeneic MSC therapy, it should be done using time points that would allow detection of antibody responses.

DISCLOSURES

None.

REFERENCES

1. Salz RO, Elliott CRB, Zuffa T, et al. Treatment of racehorse superficial digital flexor tendonitis: a comparison of stem cell treatments to controlled exercise rehabilitation in 213 cases. Equine Vet J 2023. https://doi.org/10.1111/EVJ.13922.
2. Smith RKW, et al. Beneficial effects of autologous bone marrow-derived mesenchymal stem cells in naturally occurring tendinopathy. PLoS One 2013;8.
3. Prządka P, et al. The role of mesenchymal stem cells (MSCs) in veterinary medicine and their use in musculoskeletal disorders. Biomolecules 2021;11.
4. Ankrum J, Ong J, Karp J. Mesenchymal stem cells: immune evasive, not immune privileged. Nat Biotechnol 2014;252–60.
5. Hoogduijn M, Lombardo E. Mesenchymal stromal cells anno 2019: dawn of the therapeutic era? Concise review. Stem Cells Transl Med 2019;1126–34.
6. Caplan H, et al. Mesenchymal stromal cell therapeutic delivery: translational challenges to clinical application. Front Immunol 2019;1645.
7. Barry F. MSC therapy for osteoarthritis: an unfinished story. J Orthop Res 2019;1229–35.
8. Jevotovsky D, Alfonso A, Einhorn T, et al. Osteoarthritis and stem cell therapy in humans: a systematic review. Osteoarthritis Cartilage 2018;711–29.
9. Spaas JH, et al. Chondrogenic priming at reduced cell density enhances cartilage adhesion of equine allogeneic MSCs: a loading sensitive phenomenon in an organ culture study with 180 explants. Cell Physiol Biochem 2015;37:651–65.
10. Barrachina L, et al. Assessment of effectiveness and safety of repeat administration of proinflammatory primed allogeneic mesenchymal stem cells in an equine model of chemically induced osteoarthritis. BMC Vet Res 2018;14.

11. Cassano JM, Fortier LA, Hicks RB, et al. Equine mesenchymal stromal cells from different tissue sources display comparable immune-related gene expression profiles in response to interferon gamma (IFN)-γ. Vet Immunol Immunopathol 2018;202:25–30.
12. Caplan AI, Hariri R. Body management: mesenchymal stem cells control the internal regenerator. Stem Cells Transl Med 2015;4:695–701.
13. Caplan AI. Mesenchymal stem cells: time to change the name. Stem Cells Transl Med 2017;6:1445–51.
14. Avella CS, et al. Ultrasonographic assessment of the superficial digital flexor tendons of National Hunt racehorses in training over two racing seasons. Equine Vet J 2009;41:449–54.
15. Williams RB, Harkins LS, Hammond CJ, et al. Racehorse injuries, clinical problems and fatalities recorded on British racecourses from flat racing and National Hunt racing during 1996, 1997 and 1998. Equine Vet J 2001;33:478–86.
16. Goodship AE, Birch HL, Wilson AM. The pathobiology and repair of tendon and ligament injury. Vet Clin N Am Equine Pract 1994;10:323–49.
17. Clegg PD, Pinchbeck GL. Evidence-based medicine and stem cell therapy: how do we know such technologies are safe and efficacious? Vet Clin N Am Equine Pract 2011;27:373–82.
18. Godwin EE, Young NJ, Dudhia J, et al. Implantation of bone marrow-derived mesenchymal stem cells demonstrates improved outcome in horses with overstrain injury of the superficial digital flexor tendon. Equine Vet J 2012;44:25–32.
19. Dyson SJ. Medical management of superficial digital flexor tendonitis: a comparative study in 219 horses (1992-2000). Equine Vet J 2004;36:415–9.
20. Alves AGL, et al. Cell-based therapies for tendon and ligament injuries. Vet Clin N Am Equine Pract 2011;27:315–33.
21. Herthel DJ. Enhanced suspensory ligament healing in 100 horses by stem cells and other bone marrow components. AAEP proceedings 2001;47:319.
22. Smith RKW, Korda M, Blunn GW, et al. Isolation and implantation of autologous equine mesenchymal stem cells from bone marrow into the superficial digital flexor tendon as a potential novel treatment. Equine Vet J 2003;35:99–102.
23. Smith RKW. Mesenchymal stem cell therapy for equine tendinopathy. Disabil Rehabil 2008;30:1752–8.
24. Wike MM, Nydam DV, Nixon AJ. Enhanced early chondrogenesis in articular defects following arthroscopic mesenchymal stem cell implantation in an equine model. J Orthop Res 2007;25:913–25.
25. Van Loon VJF, Scheffer CJW, Genn HJ, et al. Clinical follow-up of horses treated with allogeneic equine mesenchymal stem cells derived from umbilical cord blood for different tendon and ligament disorders. Vet Q 2014;34:92–7.
26. Pacini S, et al. Suspension of bone marrow-derived undifferentiated mesenchymal stromal cells for repair of superficial digital flexor tendon in race horses. Tissue Eng 2007;13:2949–55.
27. Caron, J. P., Genovese, R. L., Ross, M. W. & Dyson, S. J. Principles and practices of joint disease treatment. in Diagnosis and Management of Lameness in the Horse 572-591. (2003).
28. Broeckx S, et al. Regenerative therapies for equine degenerative joint disease: a preliminary study. PLoS One 2014;9.
29. Berg LC, et al. Chondrogenic potential of mesenchymal stromal cells derived from equine bone marrow and umbilical cord blood. Vet Comp Orthop Traumatol 2009;22:363–70.

30. Frisbie DD, Kisiday JD, Kawcak CE, et al. Evaluation of adipose-derived stromal vascular fraction or bone marrow-derived mesenchymal stem cells for treatment of osteoarthritis. J Orthop Res 2009;27:1675–80.
31. McIlwraith CW, et al. Evaluation of intra-articular mesenchymal stem cells to augment healing of microfractured chondral defects. Arthroscopy 2011;27:1552–61.
32. Ferris DJ, et al. Clinical outcome after intra-articular administration of bone marrow derived mesenchymal stem cells in 33 horses with stifle injury. Vet Surg 2014;43:255–65.
33. Nicpoń J, Marycz K, Grzesiak J. Therapeutic effect of adipose-derived mesenchymal stem cell injection in horses suffering from bone spavin. Pol J Vet Sci 2013;16:753–4.
34. Mariñas-Pardo L, et al. Allogeneic adipose-derived mesenchymal stem cells (Horse Allo 20) for the treatment of osteoarthritis-associated lameness in horses: characterization, safety, and efficacy of intra-articular treatment. Stem Cells Dev 2018;27:1147–60.
35. Available at: https://www.ema.europa.eu/en/medicines/veterinary/EPAR/horse-allo-20 .
36. Magri C, et al. Comparison of efficacy and safety of single versus repeated intra-articular injection of allogeneic neonatal mesenchymal stem cells for treatment of osteoarthritis of the metacarpophalangeal/metatarsophalangeal joint in horses: a clinical pilot study. PLoS One 2019;14.
37. Rowland AL, et al. Cross-matching of allogeneic mesenchymal stromal cells eliminates recipient immune targeting. Stem Cells Transl Med 2021;10:694–710.
38. Pradera, A. Efficacy and safety study of allogeneic equine umbilical cord derived mesenchymal stem cells (EUC-MSCs) for the treatment of clinical symptomatology associated (Dissertation). (2019).
39. Broeckx S, et al. Allogenic mesenchymal stem cells as a treatment for equine degenerative joint disease: a pilot study. Curr Stem Cell Res Ther 2014;9:497–503.
40. Broeckx SY, et al. Equine allogeneic chondrogenic induced mesenchymal stem cells are an effective treatment for degenerative joint disease in horses. Stem Cells Dev 2019;28:410–22.
41. Van Hecke L, et al. Repeated intra-articular administration of equine allogeneic peripheral blood-derived mesenchymal stem cells does not induce a cellular and humoral immune response in horses. Vet Immunol Immunopathol 2021;239.
42. Hare JM, et al. Comparison of allogeneic vs autologous bone marrow–derived mesenchymal stem cells delivered by transendocardial injection in patients with ischemic cardiomyopathy: the POSEIDON randomized trial. JAMA 2012;308:2369–79.
43. Le Blanc K, et al. Mesenchymal stem cells for treatment of steroid-resistant, severe, acute graft-versus-host disease: a phase II study. Lancet 2008;371:1579–86.
44. Yi H, Wang Y, Liang Q, et al. Preclinical and clinical amelioration of bone fractures with mesenchymal stromal cells: a systematic review and meta-analysis. Cell Transplant 2022;31.
45. Klein CE, et al. Comparative results of 3 treatments for medial femoral condyle subchondral cystic lesions in Thoroughbred racehorses. Vet Surg 2022;51:455–63.
46. Campbell TM, et al. Mesenchymal stem cell alterations in bone marrow lesions in patients with hip osteoarthritis. Arthritis Rheumatol 2016;68:1648–59.

47. Fellows CR, et al. Characterisation of a divergent progenitor cell sub-populations in human osteoarthritic cartilage: the role of telomere erosion and replicative senescence. Sci Rep 2017;7.
48. Harman RM, et al. Single-cell RNA sequencing of equine mesenchymal stromal cells from primary donor-matched tissue sources reveals functional heterogeneity in immune modulation and cell motility. Stem Cell Res Ther 2020;11.
49. García-Sancho J, Sánchez A, Vega A, et al. Influence of HLA matching on the efficacy of allogeneic mesenchymal stromal cell therapies for osteoarthritis and degenerative disc disease. Transplant Direct 2017;3:E205.
50. Reinders ME, et al. Safety of allogeneic bone marrow derived mesenchymal stromal cell therapy in renal transplant recipients: the Neptune study. J Transl Med 2015;13.
51. Berglund AK, Fortier LA, Antczak DF, et al. Immunoprivileged no more: measuring the immunogenicity of allogeneic adult mesenchymal stem cells. Stem Cell Res Ther 2017;8.
52. Cequier A, et al. The immunomodulation-immunogenicity balance of equine mesenchymal stem cells (MSCs) is differentially affected by the immune cell response depending on inflammatory licensing and major histocompatibility complex (MHC) compatibility. Front Vet Sci 2022;9:957153.
53. Pezzanite LM, et al. Equine allogeneic bone marrow-derived mesenchymal stromal cells elicit antibody responses in vivo. Stem Cell Res Ther 2015;6.
54. Berglund AK, Schnabel LV. Allogeneic major histocompatibility complex-mismatched equine bone marrow-derived mesenchymal stem cells are targeted for death by cytotoxic anti-major histocompatibility complex antibodies. Equine Vet J 2017;49:539–44.
55. Joswig AJ, et al. Repeated intra-articular injection of allogeneic mesenchymal stem cells causes an adverse response compared to autologous cells in the equine model. Stem Cell Res Ther 2017;8:42.
56. Zangi L, et al. Direct imaging of immune rejection and memory induction by allogeneic mesenchymal stromal cells. Stem Cell 2009;27:2865–74.
57. Giri J, Galipeau J. Mesenchymal stromal cell therapeutic potency is dependent upon viability, route of delivery, and immune match. Blood Adv 2020;4:1987–97.
58. Tallmadge RL, Campbell JA, Miller DC, et al. Analysis of MHC class I genes across horse MHC haplotypes. Immunogenetics 2010;62:159–72.
59. Álvaro-Gracia JM, et al. Intravenous administration of expanded allogeneic adipose-derived mesenchymal stem cells in refractory rheumatoid arthritis (Cx611): results of a multicentre, dose escalation, randomised, single-blind, placebo-controlled phase Ib/IIa clinical trial. Ann Rheum Dis 2017;76:196–202.
60. Rowland AL, Burns ME, Levine GJ, et al. Preparation technique affects recipient immune targeting of autologous mesenchymal stem cells. Front Vet Sci 2021;8.
61. Arzi B, et al. Therapeutic efficacy of fresh, autologous mesenchymal stem cells for severe refractory gingivostomatitis in cats. Stem Cells Transl Med 2016;5:75–86.
62. Owens SD, Kol A, Walker NJ, et al. Allogeneic mesenchymal stem cell treatment induces specific alloantibodies in horses. Stem Cell Int 2016;2016.
63. Gershwin LJ, Netherwood KA, Norris MS, et al. Equine IgE responses to non-viral vaccine components. Vaccine 2012;30:7615–20.
64. Simkin PA, Pizzorno JE. Synovial permeability in rheumatoid arthritis. Arthritis Rheum 1979;22:689–96.
65. Levick JR. Permeability of rheumatoid and normal human synovium to specific plasma proteins. Arthritis Rheum 1981;24:1550–60.

66. Berner D, et al. Longitudinal cell tracking and simultaneous monitoring of tissue regeneration after cell treatment of natural tendon disease by low-field magnetic resonance imaging. Stem Cell Int 2016;2016.
67. Galipeau J, Sensébé L. Mesenchymal stromal cells: clinical challenges and therapeutic opportunities. Cell Stem Cell 2018;22:824–33.
68. Mirghaderi SP, et al. Cell therapy efficacy and safety in treating tendon disorders: a systemic review of clinical studies. J Exp Orthop 2022;9.
69. Copp G, Robb KP, Viswanathan S. Culture-expanded mesenchymal stromal cell therapy: does it work in knee osteoarthritis? A pathway to clinical success. Cell Mol Immunol 2023;20.

Advances in Imaging Techniques to Guide Therapies and Monitor Response to the Treatment of Musculoskeletal Injuries

Caitlyn R. Horne, DVM, DACVSMR*, Sara Tufts, DVM

KEYWORDS

• Horse • Musculoskeletal • Diagnostic imaging • Ultrasound
• Magnetic resonance imaging • Computed tomography • Nuclear scintigraphy
• Radiography

KEY POINTS

- Diagnostic imaging modalities should be selected based on each individual case depending on the anatomic location, possible differentials, and type of information needed to select a treatment plan or monitor an existing lesion.
- Each imaging modalities used in the horse (ultrasound, radiography, nuclear scintigraphy, MRI, CT, and PET) has its own unique strengths and weaknesses therefore multiple modalities are frequently used in conjunction with each other.
- Recheck or continued monitoring with diagnostic imaging aids in better disease understanding, progression, and treatment selection.
- A complete diagnostic imaging workup provides the most accurate and complete diagnosis and can then be used as a tool to increase precise targeted treatment leading to more efficacious treatment.

INTRODUCTION

Continual advancements in diagnostic imaging have allowed for more accurate and complete diagnoses of injuries in the performance horse. The use of several different imaging tools has further allowed the equine sports medicine clinician to more carefully direct treatment options, monitor response to therapy, and guide rehabilitation recommendations. The advancements in diagnostic imaging and novel treatment

North Carolina State University College of Veterinary Medicine, 1060 William Moore Drive, Raleigh, NC 27607, USA
* Corresponding author.
E-mail address: cdreddin@ncsu.edu

Vet Clin Equine 39 (2023) 489–501
https://doi.org/10.1016/j.cveq.2023.06.001
vetequine.theclinics.com
0749-0739/23/

options have led to the improvement in the overall prognosis of many injuries that affect the horse and their performance. The purpose of this section is to review the advancements made in diagnostic imaging of the horse and to aid the practitioner in the selection of the appropriate modality and how best to use them to guide treatment and monitoring decisions (**Fig. 1**).

DIAGNOSTIC IMAGING MODALITIES

Ultrasound

Ultrasound remains a practical, non-invasive, and easily accessible imaging technique for the real-time evaluation of soft tissue structures, peripheral margins of osseous structures, and accessible areas of articular cartilage. Traditional gray scale, or B-mode, ultrasonography has been the mainstay for decades for the diagnosis and monitoring of tendon and ligament injuries. Transverse and longitudinal planes are used to evaluate the size, shape, echogenicity, and overall fiber pattern of the different structures. Measurements of the cross-sectional area of the structure(s) involved and characterization of lesion(s) in the transverse plane is important to provide baseline measurements of the injury. It is also important to document the proximal to distal extent of lesion and to subjectively evaluate the appearance of the fiber pattern. Establishing the characteristics of a lesion in both cross-section and longitudinal is critical for diagnosis, treatment selection, and as future monitoring parameters. Serial use of diagnostic ultrasound is a powerful tool to document and monitor the progression of a lesion. However, it is important to recognize a limitation of ultrasound to depict the appearance of healed tendons or ligaments before they are potentially histologically healed. This should be considered when making treatment and monitoring decisions and explains the need for more in-depth imaging techniques.

While ultrasound is commonly used as a first-line imaging technique it important to also recognize its utility as a monitoring tool following more advanced imaging. Ultrasound is a more affordable and convenient recheck imaging modality following an MRI or CT examination and therefore should be viewed as complementary to these more advanced modalities.

Determination of acute versus chronic

Color or power Doppler ultrasonography is newer ultrasound techniques that are becoming more widely available on most ultrasound machines. While color Doppler measures the velocity and direction of blood flow, Power Doppler looks rather at the total strength of the returning echoes, therefore making it a more sensitive measure of neovascularization. Microvasculature is present throughout the inflammatory, proliferative, and reparative phases of healing. Once the remodeling phase begins, vascular flow should subside as the tissue begins to fibrose.[1] Therefore, Doppler

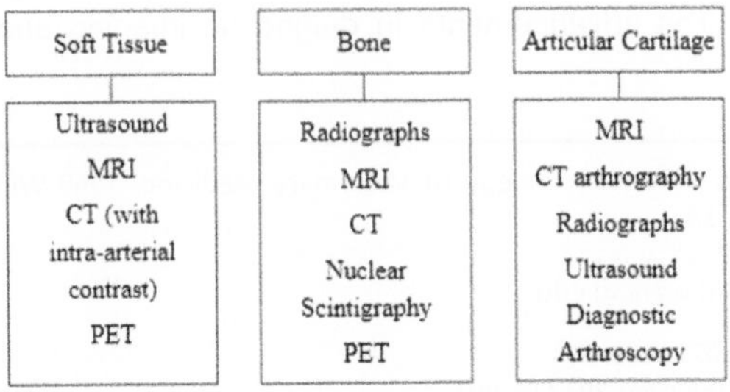

Fig. 1. Overview of diagnostic imaging modality selection based on tissue type.

has the potential to be able to indicate approximately the stage of healing of a soft tissue injury. Currently, there is limited research on using Doppler in the horse. One equine study assessed vascular flow with power Doppler after surgically creating SDF tendinitis and treating them with PRP. The study found increased blood flow out to 23 weeks in the treated limbs.[2] Another study looked at suspensory ligament branches in 13 horses that showed microvasculature flow was present in both acute and chronic lesions but not in normal branches. These results were not correlated with clinical soundness.[3] In a human study looking at power Doppler flow in achilles tendons, neovascularization was present in the region of structural tendon change in all painful tendons, but flow was not present in any of the pain-free normal tendons.[4]

When using Doppler it is important to recognize operator variability may affect the results such as weight bearing versus non-weight bearing, size of color box, and pressure applied. Currently, the authors use power doppler in clinical cases to help determine the clinical relevance of a lesion but more importantly in conjunction with routine ultrasound assessment of an injury to help guide decisions pertaining to the stage of healing of an injury (**Fig. 2**). Serial use of Doppler assessment of blood flow may be helpful to subjectively determine the stage of healing and how that may influence the degree of activity of an injury. However, further investigation is still required to determine if the pattern and degree of neovascularization can be used to assess the stage of healing and the efficacy of different therapies and rehabilitation decisions.

Elastography is an additional technique that has been evaluated in the horse in hopes to have another technique to monitor healing of tendons and ligaments. Elastography measures tissue strain by applying external manual compression with the ultrasound transducer. A color mapping of the evaluated area is provided showing soft

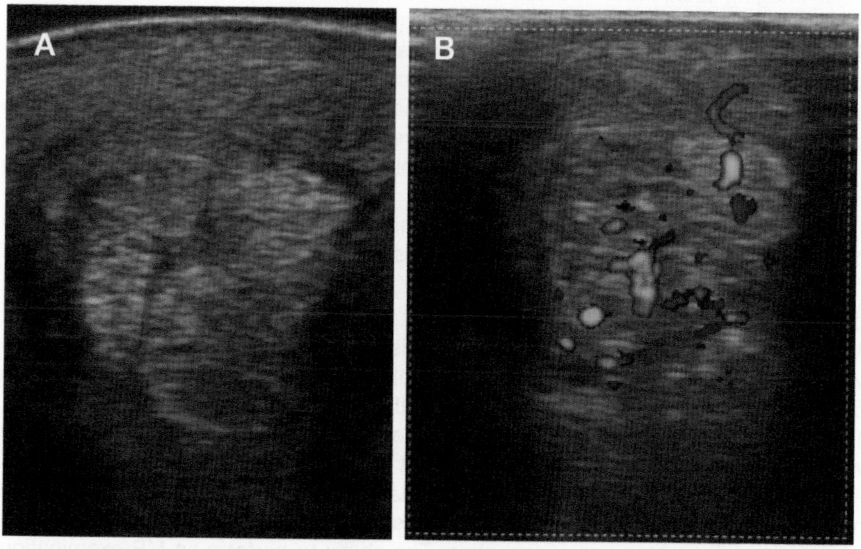

Fig. 2. Corresponding ultrasound images of a hind medial suspensory ligament branch. (*A*) This is a gray-scale image in a weight-bearing patient showing mild to moderate fiber pattern irregularity centrally and mild to moderate periligamentous soft tissue thickening. (*B*) Is the same region of the suspensory branch using power Doppler, on non-weight bearing examination, showing mild to moderate neovascularization within the area of abnormal fiber pattern. Image courtesy of Dr Sarah Gold, DVM, ACVSMR.

or damaged tendon as one color and harder or normal tendon being another color. In a study assessing the elasticity of distal limb injuries identified with magnetic resonance imaging or B-mode ultrasonography, acute lesions were softer and more hypoechoic compared to stiffer and more hyperechoic chronic lesions.[5] This too could provide another useful tool for monitoring lesion progression.

Ultrasound-guided techniques

Real-time imaging makes ultrasound the ideal tool to accurately guide interventional techniques such as the injection of diagnostic anesthetics, intra-articular medications, and regenerative therapies. Ultrasound-guided techniques have been described for many anatomic locations with improved accuracy for the placement of the injectate over blind approaches. It is important to note that the skill and ease in the use of ultrasound in some of these techniques is still very operator-dependent and sterile technique must be maintained.

Additional ultrasound advancements (pocket size ultrasound)

Ultrasound technology is quickly advancing making this a tool that is becoming more widely available due to smaller sizes and more affordable pricing than traditional ultrasounds. A study compared images from a traditional versus pocket size ultrasound in several clinical situations including musculoskeletal ultrasound. They found that while a difference in image quality is evident from the traditional ultrasound, the pocket sized ultrasound still would have likely been adequate for decision making.[6]

Limitations

Ultrasonography has many limitations that need to be recognized. The quality of the image is directly related to the operator, the equipment, and the anatomic area being examined. This imaging tool is influenced by the skill of the operator more than any other imaging technique. The operator is responsible for positioning and steering the sound beam as well as determining the equipment settings during image acquisition. Artifacts are easily produced and can create inaccuracies in the image, which can significantly compromise interpretation. Artifacts most often involve operator error and an assortment of sound-tissue interactions that may or may not be controllable. One common but easily correctable artifact is created by inadequate skin preparation. Inadequate skin prep leads to poor transmission of sound and a corresponding dark image.

Ultrasound is limited when it comes to visualizing structures within the hoof capsule making MRI still necessary to rule out soft tissue injuries in the foot.

Magnetic Resonance Imaging

MRI is considered the gold standard for the distal limb of the horse. MRI not only provides structural but physiologic information about the soft tissues and bones of the distal limb of the horse but can demonstrate the presence of inflammation or edema. The increasing use of MRI in the horse has allowed us to identify soft tissue and bone injuries not previously recognized and to treat injuries more precisely and accurately.

As technology continues to advance, MRI has become more widely available to the horse. Increasing numbers of equine facilities have installed low-field MRIs (0.27 T) which allows for a standing examination. The ability to perform an MR examination of the distal limb without the need for general anesthesia has increased the willingness of many owners to have MR performed and to allow recheck examination(s). The ability to perform serial MRI examinations can lead to a better understanding of these disease processes, assist us in making better therapeutic decisions, and allows us to monitor lesion and treatment progression.

On the other side of the MRI spectrum, continued advancements in MRI technology have allowed many facilities to install even stronger magnets than the traditional high-field magnets that were 1 T (T) or 1.5 T to now 3T magnets. With this advancement comes better image quality and more efficient scanning times. As the installation of these magnets is still relatively recent there is undoubtedly more information to come with more research being performed on these magnets that may teach us even more.

Low-field versus high-field magnetic resonance imaging

It is important to recognize the differences between low-field and high-field MRI as they are critical to case selection. A low-field magnet has the advantage of being a standing procedure, however patient compliance is still imperative, with even swaying from sedation or weight shifting altering ideal image acquisition (**Fig. 3**). Therefore the time it takes to acquire a standing examination can vary greatly depending on the patient, imaging protocol, and area of interest, with the proximal limb being more severely affected by motion artifact. A high-field MRI does require general anesthesia which is not without risk. However, due to the horse being anesthetized, image acquisition can be more routinely performed within a set time and without the risk of image quality being altered by patient motion.

The main advantage of a high-field MRI is the image resolution (**Fig. 4**). The increased structural detail obtained with a high-field magnet is far superior to a low-field magnet. This makes a high-field magnet a better choice for cases with more subtle lesions or in low-grade lameness where disease pathology is often more mild. It is important to note that while high-field MRI is superior for imaging articular cartilage in the horse, there still remains limitations of MRI when imaging cartilage and sequence selection is imperative. Multiple studies have compared different sequences, the use of intra articular contrast, but yet there continues to be limitations in visualizing subtle articular cartilage lesions especially in certain joints with thin cartilage such as the fetlock.[7,8] Hopefully this is an area that the 3T high-field magnets prove to be beneficial.

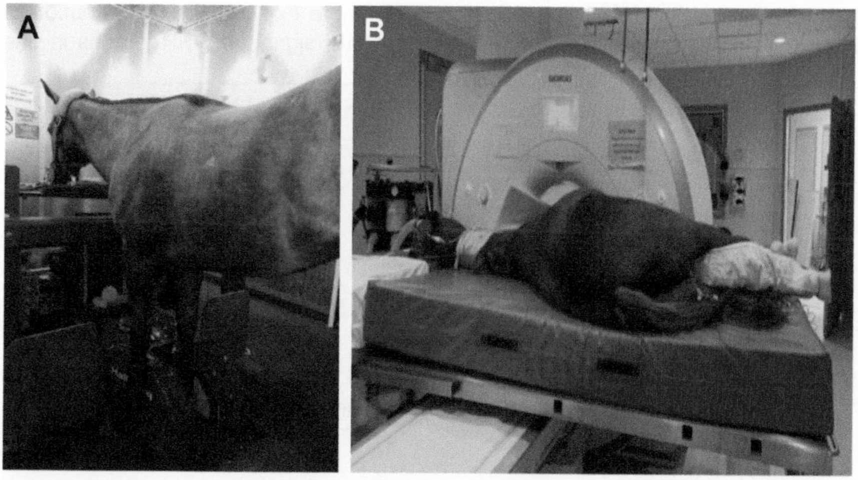

Fig. 3. (*A*) The image shows a horse having a standing MRI examination of the foot region using a low-field magnet (0.27 T). (*B*) The image shows the positioning of a horse under general anesthesia for a forelimb MRI scan using in high-field (3T) magnet. Image courtesy of Dr. Sarah Gold, DVM, ACVSMR.

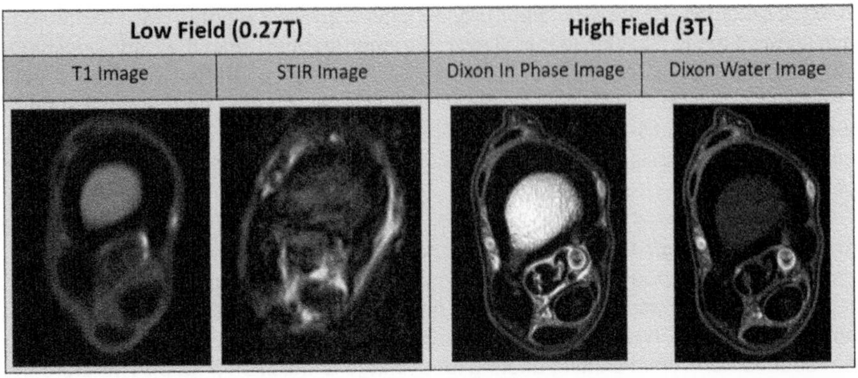

Fig. 4. Representative images from transverse sequences of a normal hind proximal suspensory ligament using a low-field magnet (0.27 T) compared to a high-field (3T) magnet. This highlights the superior image resolution when using a high-field MRI.

Determination of acute versus chronic

On MRI, different sequences of the same anatomic location can have varying signal intensities and are used to determine if a lesion is potentially acute or chronic. An acute or chronic lesion will be apparent on T1-weighted (T1-w) images with chronic lesions persisting for an unknown length of time or potentially forever. Whereas an acute lesion will have signal on T2-w images and slowly decrease in signal throughout the stages of healing (**Fig. 5**). This was shown in a study that looked at surgically created lesions in the superficial digital flexor tendon where it was difficult to see the lesions at 12 weeks on both T2-w and STIR images (using a 1.5 T magnet) and resolution of signal was seen on T2-w images[9] (see **Fig. 5**). It is important to note that this can be more complex. While acute lesions in theory should gradually improve on STIR sequences, in a study looking at acute and chronic naturally occurring deep digital flexor tendon lesions, some lesions persisted on the STIR sequences, which was correlated on histopathology with core necrosis. While cases where the signal improved on STIR sequences but remained on T2-w images, the lesion was found to be consistent with fibroplasia on histopath.[10] It is also important to note that the clinical resolution of lameness was correlated with the resolution of MRI signal on STIR images in one

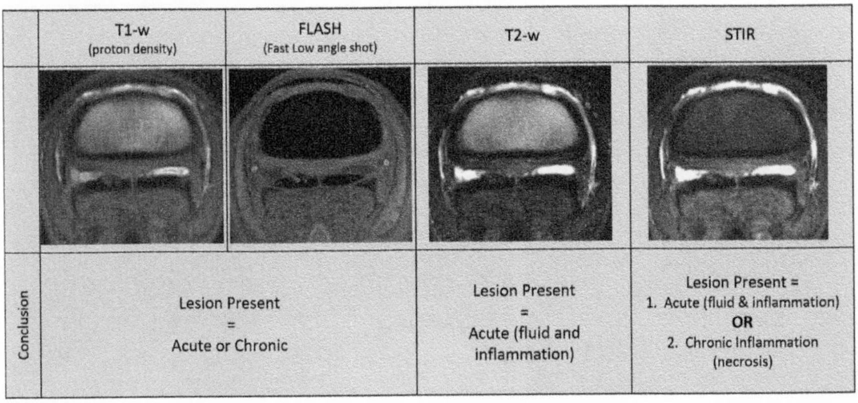

T1-w
(proton density)
FLASH
(Fast Low angle shot)
T2-w
STIR
Conclusion
Lesion Present
=
Acute or Chronic
Lesion Present
=
Acute (fluid and inflammation)
Lesion Present =
1. Acute (fluid & inflammation)
OR
2. Chronic Inflammation (necrosis)

Fig. 5. MRI images of a case with a lesion within the deep digital flexor tendon on different MRI sequences and what the conclusion of the lesion being present on that sequence would mean.

study.[11] The best way to still confirm the activity of a lesion or progression is by performing a recheck MRI at a specified/designated time period based on the lesion type and expected progression timeline.

Additional factors that affect treatment decisions

Clinical examination and diagnostic analgesia are necessary to localize a lameness to a specific region. The use of MRI in the evaluation of these regions can be extremely useful to examine the complex anatomy of these specific locations. Defining whether soft tissue or bone is involved can influence the type of therapy that is most appropriate. In regions such as the proximal suspensory ligament (forelimb and hindlimb) it is critical to determine the degree of ligament and bone involvement when making therapeutic decisions. But most notably in the hindlimb, it is also important to rule out adjacent structures that may be involved. The distal hock joints may also be involved or can present with an overlap in the effects of diagnostic anesthesia. In addition, the foot may have deep digital flexor tendon, navicular bone, navicular bursa, and the impar ligament involvement. While all may be involved with navicular disease the degree of involvement of each structure may greatly change therapeutic decisions and monitoring strategies.

Limitations

Currently, MRI examination is still limited to the distal limb in both high and low-field MRIs examinations. In an average-sized horse, the distal limb from the tip of the foot to the carpus/proximal metacarpus and tarsus/proximal metatarsus can be imaged in the forelimb and hindlimb respectively (this is influenced by the size of the horse and the size of the aperture of the magnet). There is variability in every examination based on these parameters. Some high-field MRIs with large bore apertures are capable of doing skulls and cranial necks. Some low-field systems are capable of doing the stifle region with the horse under anesthesia.

Image acquisition time is heavily dependent on the field strength of the MR. While image acquisition time may be shorter with high-field magnets, time constraints associated with the duration of anesthesia may limit the acquisition of a complete study of both limbs felt to be necessary for comparison between limbs. Due to prolonged scan times MRI requires that the region of interest to be well localized with diagnostic anesthesia beforehand. Acquiring images of the opposite limb is ideal to confirm abnormalities versus normal variation or clinical significance of lesions found.

Computed Tomography Scan

CT has been utilized in veterinary medicine since the early 1990s and, until more recently, has been an imaging modality requiring general anesthesia. CT provides rapid acquisition of a cross-sectional data set with its strength being osseous structures. Cross-sectional imaging eliminates anatomic superimposition that can greatly improve the diagnostic utility/capabilities of CT imaging particularly when dealing with complex anatomy or pathology associated with areas such as the skull, tarsus, or fractures. CT can provide a 3D rendering of an area which can significantly improve the visualization of complex pathologies or assist in surgical planning. Recent advancements in CT design have allowed more portable systems that allow some machines to be moved from one room to another. CTs have frequently been utilized for pre-surgical planning but now with the increased portability they can be utilized as an intraoperative tool.

A significant recent advancement in CT imaging comes in the form of a larger aperture which allows the standing sedated horse to place its head and the cranial cervical area within the bore of the CT.[12,13] Many different CT systems are available that can be utilized for standing examinations but may require other equipment such as lifts or specific room design including a pit. The ease of performing a standing examination, especially with the short image acquisition time, has encouraged the availability of CT in a number of different academic and private practice facilities improving the investigation of clinical cases.

Some of these newer CT scanners with the wider bore system now provide the capability to image areas that were previously not possible such as the stifle, caudal neck, and elbow.[14] CT of the cervical spine with or without cervical myelography is becoming more widely used and is likely going to change the way that we understand and treat cervical spine disease.[15,16] These new imaging capabilities allow us to more accurately diagnose areas of pathology and in turn better select therapeutic options.

It is important to recognize CT has limitations when it comes to imaging soft tissue structures due to inferior contrast resolution when compared to MRI. This makes it more difficult to differentiate between soft tissue structures or between articular cartilage and joint fluid on CT. However, the use of CT arthrography has been used more widely in the horse with reports of this technique in the stifle, carpus, fetlock, and distal interphalangeal joint. This technique provides better contrast within the joint to better visualize intra articular structures such as soft tissue, or defects in articular cartilage and subchondral bone. CT has the advantage over MRI in being able to evaluate the entire joint margin in one scan in comparison to MRI where the joint is best visualized when images are acquired perpendicular to the joint space. There has been mixed evidence whether this technique is superior to MRI in visualizing intra-articular abnormalities; regardless, it appears to have comparable sensitivity and specificity and is another useful tool, especially in anatomic locations that may be limited with MRI.[8,17–19]

Determination of acute versus chronic

CT has historically lacked physiologic information. Multiple studies have now demonstrated the utility of arterial contrast CT to assess for the neovascularization of lesions.[20,21] This is an important advancement in this imaging modality to assist in making therapeutic decisions based on the degree of remodeling of a lesion. Arterial contrast CT can help to determine the degree of vascular ingrowth, which may determine how some therapies are administered or what therapies are selected.

Limitations

Imaging of different anatomic locations is still dependent on the machine, bore size, and can be influenced by the size of the horse. Standing examinations in the horse are limited and are based on the machine and setup but can include the skull, cervical spine, and distal limbs up to the carpus and tarsus.

Like radiography, it is still important to consider radiation exposure to the patient and personnel performing the examination. Strategic room designs can prove to be helpful in decreasing the radiation exposure to staff while still keeping the patient safely restrained.

Positron Emission Tomography

Positron emission tomography (PET) is a growing imaging modality in the equine industry. PET is a type of nuclear medicine that is able to provide more specific lesion localization than the traditional nuclear scintigraphy (or bone scan). This is achieved by providing both higher spatial resolution and is displayed as a cross-sectional imaging in comparison to the traditional scintigraphy that depends on orthogonal views.

Like traditional scintigraphy, PET uses a radiolabeled tracer molecule that is injected intravenously which is then distributed via vascular flow. Areas of increased uptake represent a change in the biologic process, dependent on the tracer used. When looking for osseous abnormalities, the PET tracer used is ^{18}F-sodium fluoride (NaF). ^{18}F-NaF goes to areas of osteoblastic activity being incorporated into the hydroxyapatite crystals, therefore making it a good marker for bone turnover.[22] When looking for soft tissue lesions ^{18}Fluorine-fluorodeoxyglucose (^{18}F-FDG) is used which accumulates in areas of altered glucose metabolism. Therefore, increased areas of uptake indicate more metabolically active areas. Given PET is depicting functional information it is best to pair it with the structural information given either by CT or MRI. Additionally, not all changes seen on other imaging modalities may be seen on PET nor is something seen on PET always apparent on other imaging modalities.[22,23]

Due to the sensitivity of PET scanning, it has been utilized for bone remodeling/change in the racehorse population. In a study looking at fetlocks in Thoroughbred racehorses, PET identified stress lesions in locations where catastrophic breakdown injuries occur, such as the palmar metacarpal condyles and proximal sesamoid bones. These stress lesions were not always identified on other imaging modalities.[22] While a better understanding is still needed of what constitutes a normal adaptive stress remodeling secondary to training to one that increases the risk for catastrophic breakdown. This imaging modality shows promise in the prevention of catastrophic breakdown injuries.

Given this is such a new imaging modality in the horse, more research and increased use in clinical cases will hopefully lead to a better understanding of what positive PET findings indicate and what lesions we may have been missing on other imaging modalities.

PET was recently validated for use in the evaluation of the distal limb in the standing horse including the carpus, fetlock, and foot. Image acquisition is relatively short with the recommended scan time for most fetlocks being 4 minutes.[24] The ability to use this modality in the standing horse, with a very quick scan time (in comparison to MRI) will likely only increase its availability and clinical use in the horse.

Determination of acute versus chronic

An important benefit of PET scanning is the ability to tell if a lesion is active or inactive. This could be extremely helpful in the sport horse when selecting therapies and designing rehabilitation programs. While MRI is the superior imaging modality for soft tissue injuries it remains unclear as to its reliability in determining how active a lesion is. As PET is measuring the metabolic activity of soft tissue lesions, in theory the lesion must be in the active state to be apparent on the scan. A study was performed using PET to evaluate deep digital flexor tendinopathy in 8 horses and compared these findings to CT (both with and without arterial contrast) and low-field MRI. When comparing PET to CT and MRI it most closely correlated with what were thought to be active lesions in those modalities. In CT these were images with arterial contrast and in MRI it was the T2-weighted images. In contrast, the images in those modalities that are likely to show more chronic lesions, such as the precontrast CT and T1-weighted images on MRI, correlated less with the PET scan images.[23]

In addition, PET scanning has the capability to quantify the degree of uptake (SUVmax - maximal standardized uptake values) of a certain lesion making this modality a potentially great resource for recheck examinations and therapeutic monitoring. This will hopefully lead to this imaging tool being able to grade lesion severity and then potentially track lesion progression over time.[24]

Limitations

Using PET imaging alone may prove difficult in providing exact lesion localization due to the low spatial resolution. Therefore, it is currently most useful when paired with CT images or potentially MRI images which in turn adds more cost to an overall case. In addition, performing two imaging modalities provides some inherent difficulties with pairing the images dependent on how the images were acquired.

Similar to traditional nuclear scintigraphy, image quality can be affected by poor uptake (similar to cold leg syndrome), motion (seen most notably in the standing examination), and age-related bone remodeling (with young horse's having better image quality due active bone remodeling). Again, similar to traditional nuclear scintigraphy, there are inherent difficulties that go with PET scanning such as radiation exposure. While this is similar to the amounts with bone scan, it may limit what facilities are capable of using this modality due to the associated regulations.

Nuclear Scintigraphy

Scintigraphic evaluation involves the use of a radionuclide, the most commonly used in equine practice is 99-m technichium-labeled methylene disphosphonate which is utilized specifically to detect areas of increased osseous activity. Advancements in imaging software have improved the diagnostic quality of this modality by correcting for motion artifacts produced by respiratory and standing sedation. While scintigraphy is useful in the detection of stress-related bone injury in the young training population, it can also be utilized in mature horses with a lameness that cannot be localized, behavior which limits diagnostic anesthesia, inconsistent or multi-limb lameness, and assessment of the axial skeleton. While some use scintigraphy as a screening test in the mature sport horse population it has not been shown to be a reliable use of this modality.[25] Along with osseous abnormalities, nuclear scintigraphy has also shown clinical utility in the diagnosis of distal sesamoidean (navicular) remodeling and soft tissue insertional injuries.[26]

Limitations

Major limitations to nuclear scintigraphy include the risk of radiation exposure to staff, the investment in imaging equipment and a designated space large enough to accommodate the gantry system. In order to determine the clinical relevance of nuclear scintigraphy findings, it is critical to use multimodal imaging following the procedure.

Radiology

Radiography has been a staple of equine practice for decades. The advent of digital imaging has improved the availability and use of this modality. While digital systems provide greater diagnostic utility by accounting for technique variation, they also allow instant review of the image, a critical feature for equine veterinarians. These advancements enhance decision making, treatment, and lesion monitoring within the field.

Radiograph-guided injections can be a useful tool to provide more accurate treatment placement of a needle into complex intrasynovial structures such as the navicular bursa or distal intertarsal joints. The efficient nature of digital radiology also allows for immediate therapeutic assessment such as intraoperative osseous removal, contrast radiography to confirm both placement of injectate and evaluation of synovial structure, and more precise therapeutic podiatry treatment and evaluation.

Aside from the well-recognized use of radiology to detect appendicular skeletal abnormalities, the axial skeleton may also be assessed with greater ease with newer equipment. The cervical vertebrae can be assessed with laterolateral and oblique views to assess laterality of dorsal and ventral abnormalities. In horses with

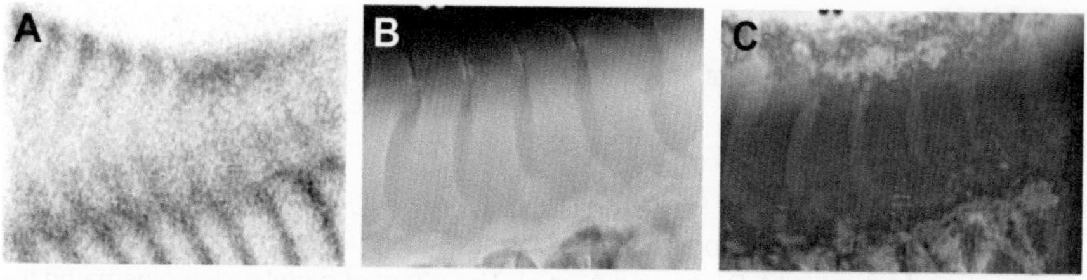

Fig. 6. (*A*) Increased radiopharmaceutical uptake visualized in the caudal thoracic dorsal spinous processes of a patient with decreased willingness to move forward under saddle. (*B*) Radiographs of this region show the impingement of the dorsal spinous processes. (*C*) Overlay of the radiographs and nuclear scintigraphy confirm ongoing osteoblastic activity in the regions of radiographic abnormalities.

thoracolumbar pain, radiographs of both the dorsal spinous processes and articular facet joints of the thoracolumbar vertebrae should be used to diagnose pathology and aid in treatment. These findings can be paired with scintigraphy and clinical signs in order to determine clinical significance[27] as seen in **Fig. 6**.

Limitations

While advancements have allowed improvements in fine bone detail of radiographs they do not provide detailed information regarding soft tissue structures or articular cartilage. Radiographs are a two dimensional image that is limited by superimposition making complex anatomic locations difficult to visualize completely. It is also important to note that radiographs do not provide physiologic information therefore with acute injuries radiographic abnormalities can lag behind clinical signs. While new machines are providing more power, there are still limitations of the equipment with increased variability in getting adequate tissue penetration in areas of increased muscle mass such as the axial skeleton (caudal cervical vertebrae, thoracolumbar articular facet joints, and pelvis).

CLINICS CARE POINTS

- Ultrasound is an important modality for monitoring lesions once diagnosed with more advanced imaging modalities such as MRI or CT as well as assisting in with more accurate treatment placement with ultrasound guided procedures.
- Understanding the pros and cons of both low field and high field MRI helps determine which cases are best suited for each as well as providing a better expectation for what information you can expect to receive depending on the magnet selected.
- PET scanners are still a new modality in the equine world and therefore it is still in the new stages of determining the clinical relevance of the information provided.
- It is important to understand the benefits and limitations with nuclear scintigraphy in the sport horse when determining how best to use it. It does not rule out soft tissue injuries in most cases and due to the lack of anatomic detail provided further imaging post scan is frequently required.

CONFLICT OF INTEREST

The author has no conflicts of interest.

DISCLOSURE

The Author has no conflicts of interest.

REFERENCES

1. Lacitignola L, Rossella S, Pasquale DL, et al. Power Doppler to investigate superficial digital flexor tendinopathy in the horse. Open Vet J 2019;9(4):317–21.
2. Bosch G, Moleman M, Barneveld A, et al. The effect of platelet-rich plasma on the neovascularization of surgically created equine superficial digital flexor tendon lesions. Scand J Med Sci Sport 2011;21(4):554–61.
3. Rabba S, Grulke S, Verwilghen D, et al. B-mode and power Doppler ultrasonography of the equine suspensory ligament branches: A descriptive study on 13 horses. Vet Radiol Ultrasound 2018;59(4). https://doi.org/10.1111/vru.12610.
4. Kristoffersen M, Öhberg L, Johnston C, et al. Neovascularisation in chronic tendon injuries detected with colour Doppler ultrasound in horse and man: Implications for research and treatment. Knee Surgery, Sport Traumatol Arthrosc 2005; 13(6):505–8.
5. Lustgarten M, Redding WR, Labens R, et al. Elastographic evaluation of naturally occurring tendon and ligament injuries of the equine distal limb. Vet Radiol Ultrasound 2015;56(6):670–9.
6. Deacon LJ, Reef VB, Leduc L, et al. Pocket-Sized Ultrasound Versus Traditional Ultrasound Images in Equine Imaging: A Pictorial Essay. J Equine Vet Sci 2021; 104:103672.
7. Werpy NM, Ho CP, Pease AP, et al. The effect of sequence selection and field strength on detection of osteochondral defects in the metacarpophalangeal joint. Vet Radiol Ultrasound 2011;52(2):154–60.
8. Porter EG, Winter MD, Sheppard BJ, et al. Correlation of Articular Cartilage Thickness Measurements made with Magentic Resonance Imaging, Magnetic Resonance Arthrography, and Computed Tomographic Arthrography with Gross Articular Cartilage Thickness in the Equine the Metacarpophalangeal Joint. Vet Radiol Ultrasound 2016;57(5):515–25.
9. Schramme M, Kerekes Z, Hunter S, et al. Mr imaging features of surgically induced core lesions in the equine superficial digital flexor tendon. Vet Radiol Ultrasound 2010;51(3):280–7.
10. Blunden A, Murray R, Dyson S. Lesions of the deep digital flexor tendon in the digit: A correlative MRI and post mortem study in control and lame horses. Equine Vet J 2009;41(1):25–33.
11. Vanel M, Olive J, Gold S, et al. Clinical significance and prognosis of deep digital flexor tendinopathy assessed over time using MRI. Vet Radiol Ultrasound 2012; 53(6):621–7.
12. Mageed M. Standing computed tomography of the equine limb using a multislice helical scanner: Technique and feasibility study. Equine Vet Educ 2022; 34(2):77–83.
13. Mathee N, Robert M, Higgerty SM, et al. Computed tomographic evaluation of the distal limb in the standing sedated horse: Technique, imaging diagnoses, feasibility, and artifacts. Vet Radiol Ultrasound 2022;1–10. https://doi.org/10.1111/vru.13182.
14. Zimmerman M, Schramme M, Barthélemy A, et al. CT is a feasible imaging technique for detecting lesions in horses with elbow lameness: A study of 139 elbows in 99 horses. Vet Radiol Ultrasound 2022;63(2):164–75.

15. Gough SL, Anderson JDC, Dixon JJ. Computed tomographic cervical myelography in horses: Technique and findings in 51 clinical cases. J Vet Intern Med 2020; 34(5):2142–51.
16. Lindgren CM, Wright L, Kristoffersen M, et al. Computed tomography and myelography of the equine cervical spine: 180 cases (2013–2018). Equine Vet Educ 2021;33(9):475–83.
17. Nelson BB, Kawcak CE, Goodrich LR, et al. Comparison Between Computed Tomographic Arthrography, Radiography, Ultrasonography, and Arthroscopy for the Diagnosis of Femorotibial Joint Disease in Western Performance Horses. Vet Radiol Ultrasound 2016;57(4):387–402.
18. Suarez Sanchez-Andrade J, Richter H, Kuhn K, et al. Comparison between magnetic resonance imaging, computed tomography, and arthrography to identify artificially induced cartilage defects of the equine carpal joints. Vet Radiol Ultrasound 2018;59(3):312–25.
19. Aßmann AD, Ohlerth S, Suárez Sánchez-Andráde J, et al. Ex vivo comparison of 3 Tesla magnetic resonance imaging and multidetector computed tomography arthrography to identify artificial soft tissue lesions in equine stifles. Vet Surg 2022;51(4):648–57.
20. Puchalski SM, Galuppo LD, Drew CP, et al. Use of contrast-enhanced computed tomography to assess angiogenesis in deep digital flexor tendonopathy in a horse. Vet Radiol Ultrasound 2009;50(3):292–7.
21. Puchalski SM, Galuppo LD, Hornof WJ, et al. Intraarterial contrast-enhanced computed tomography of the equine distal extremity. Vet Radiol Ultrasound 2007;48(1):21–9.
22. Spriet M, Espinosa-Mur P, Cissell DD, et al. 18 F-sodium fluoride positron emission tomography of the racing Thoroughbred fetlock: Validation and comparison with other imaging modalities in nine horses. Equine Vet J 2019;51(3):375–83.
23. Wilson S, Spriet M, Mur PE, et al. 18Fluorine-fluorodeoxyglucose positron emission tomography for assessment of deep digital flexor tendinopathy: An exploratory study in eight horses with comparison to CT and MRI. Vet Radiol Ultrasound 2021;62(5):610–20.
24. Spriet M, Edwards L, Arndt S, et al. Validation of a dedicated positron emission tomography scanner for imaging of the distal limb of standing horses. Vet Radiol Ultrasound 2022;63(4):469–77.
25. Quiney LE, Ireland JL, Dyson SJ. Evaluation of the diagnostic accuracy of skeletal scintigraphy in lame and poorly performing sports horses. Vet Radiol Ultrasound 2018;59(4):477–89.
26. Quiney LE, Ireland JL, Dyson SJ. Evaluation of the diagnostic accuracy of skeletal scintigraphy for the causes of front foot pain determined by magnetic resonance imaging. Vet Radiol Ultrasound 2018;59(4):490–8.
27. Zimmerman M, Dyson S, Murray R. Close, impinging and overriding spinous processes in the thoracolumbar spine: The relationship between radiological and scintigraphic findings and clinical signs. Equine Vet J 2012;44(2):178–84.

Advances in Regional Vascular Injection Techniques for the Delivery of Stem Cells to Musculoskeletal Injury Sites

Mathieu Spriet, DVM, MS, DACVR, DECVDI, DACVR-EDI[a,*],
Betsy Vaughan, DVM, DACVSMR[a],
Myra Barrett, DVM, MS, DACVR, DACVR-EDI[b],
Larry D. Galuppo, DVM, DACVS[a]

KEYWORDS

• Stem cells • Regenerative medicine • Regional limb perfusion • Intra-arterial • Tendon • Ligament • Bone

KEY POINTS

- Regional vascular injections of stem cells are pertinent for the treatment of difficult to access, extensive or multiple lesions.
- Intra-venous regional limb perfusions have limitations regarding the distribution and retention of stem cells.
- Intra-arterial injections of stem cells performed without a tourniquet appear safe and provide good distribution and retention of stem cells.
- Injection of the median artery for the front limb and the cranial tibial artery for the hind limb can be performed in standing sedated horses.

INTRODUCTION

Stem cells have been used for the treatment of various lesions in the equine distal limb.[1–3] Some of these lesions are amenable for direct injection of the stem cells, typically using ultrasound guidance,[3–5] however based on lesion location, intralesional

---

Dr M. Barrett's spouse has shares in a stem cell company.

[a] Department of Surgical and Radiological Sciences, School of Veterinary Medicine, University of California, Davis, 2112 Tupper Hall, One Shields Avenue, Davis, CA 95616, USA; [b] Department of Environmental and Radiological Health Sciences, College of Veterinary Medicine, Colorado State University, 300 West Drake Road, Fort Collins, CO 80523, USA
* Corresponding author.
E-mail address: mspriet@ucdavis.edu

https://doi.org/10.1016/j.cveq.2023.06.009

delivery is not always possible. A classic example would be lesions of the distal aspect of the deep digital flexor tendon that are difficult to reach due to the presence of the structures of the hoof. Another limitation to direct injection of stem cells in a lesion relates to multiple or extensive lesions that would require multiple injections. Concerns have also been brought with potential iatrogenic damage due to needle tracking in healthy tissues surrounding the lesion. Introduction of a needle within the superficial digital flexor tendon, as a control to laser-induced lesion in a tendinopathy model study, revealed significant tendon damage from the needle introduction itself resulting in the transection and retraction of fibers with the development of granulation tissue within the tendon.[6] A magnetic resonance imaging (MRI) tracking study demonstrated limited retention of stem cells within collagenous tendon with accumulation primarily in the surrounding fascia.[5]

For these reasons, assessing alternative ways of administrations of stem cells was considered. Vascular injections provide several possible opportunities for simpler and less invasive administrations of stem cells. Systemic injection of stem cells, through the jugular vein for example, are of limited values for musculoskeletal injuries due to the primary retention of stem cells in lungs,[7] however administration to a regional limb vessel is a promising option, especially considering the potential chemotactic homing abilities of stem cells.[8]

We will review later in discussion the different techniques that have been assessed for the administration of stem cells to lesions of the equine distal limbs, describe in further details the intra-arterial injection techniques and discuss their current clinical applications.

COMPARISON OF DIFFERENT REGIONAL VASCULAR INJECTION TECHNIQUES

Multiple techniques of vascular injections are available in the limb, these include the injection of a vein or an artery, use or not of a tourniquet and various proximal to distal sites. The use of radiolabeled stem cells has allowed scintigraphic comparison of these various techniques using research horses.

Cephalic vein regional limb perfusion was the first technique investigated in a study utilizing normal limbs.[9] Using a pneumatic tourniquet on the forearm for 30 minutes resulted in the retention of all the stem cells in the limb while the tourniquet was in place and no major departure of stem cells was observed immediately after removal of the tourniquet.[9] However only 3 of the 6 injected limbs had radioactive signal in the entire distal limb, while the other 3 limbs only had uptake in the carpal and proximal metacarpal areas. The maximal signal intensity was mostly in the area of the larger vessels (**Fig. 1**A).[9] When the study was repeated in horses with induced lesions in the superficial digital flexor tendon, the distribution and quantification of the radioactive signal was not different from the control horses.[10]

Assessment of regional limb perfusion using the median artery was also performed in the same studies with a pneumatic tourniquet on the forearm of anesthetized horses.[9,10] Radiolabeled stem cells were identified distributing through the entire distal limb in all 12 limbs injected with this technique, demonstrating a better distribution than with the cephalic vein regional limb perfusion.[9] The radioactive signal distribution followed mainly the path of the arteries. In the horses with induced superficial digital flexor tendon lesions, increased radiolabeled stem cell retention was observed in the lesion area in the 2 horses with the 10-day old lesions when compared with control horses and 3-day old lesions (**Fig. 1**B).[10] The improved distribution and increased accumulation at the lesion sites suggested the arterial regional limb perfusion was

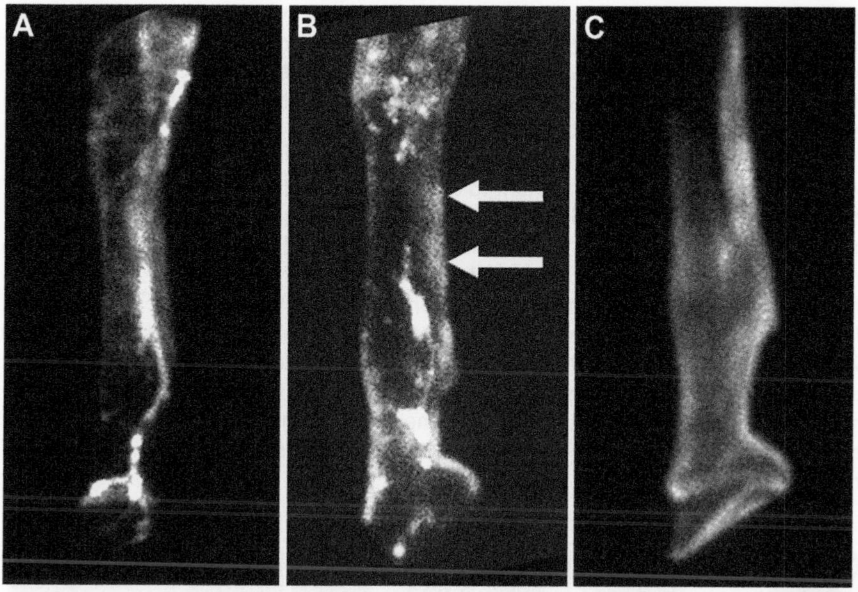

Fig. 1. Lateral scintigraphic images of the distal limb after the injection of HexamethylPropyleneAmine Oxime (HMPAO) labeled mesenchymal stem cells in horses under general anesthesia. (*A*) Regional limb perfusion of the cephalic vein with pneumatic tourniquet on the antebrachium. The radiolabeled stem cells remain primarily in the larger veins with limited distribution to the most distal aspect of the limb. (*B*) Regional limb perfusion of the median artery with a pneumatic tourniquet on the antebrachium. There is improved distal distribution when compared with the cephalic vein regional limb perfusion but the distribution remains centered on the larger vessels. The arrows indicate site of induced lesions in the superficial digital flexor tendon with evidence of stem cells accumulation. (*C*) Injection of the median artery without the use of a tourniquet. There is a more homogenous and diffuse distribution of the radiolabeled cells compared with the injections performed with a tourniquet.

more pertinent than the venous regional limb perfusion, however two out of the 12 limbs injected in the median artery developed thrombosis of the medial palmar artery resulting in lameness and skin necrosis in one of the horses.[10] The use of the tourniquet resulting in blood stasis was considered an important factor in the development of the thrombosis.[10]

In order to address the safety issue with the arterial injection of stem cells, median artery injections were performed without the use of a tourniquet.[11] A diffuse distribution of the radiolabeled cells was observed through the entire distal limb, with a more homogenous pattern, with less of a vascular distribution than when the tourniquet was used (**Fig. 1**C). Using the quantification of the radioactive signal, about half of the injected radiolabeled stem cells appeared to remain in the distal limb, despite the absence of a tourniquet.[11] The capillary bed of the distal limb appeared to have a sufficient retention power to retain a large number of stem cells. Most importantly, no evidence of thrombosis was observed on ultrasound.[11] Another objective of this study[11] was to address the unreliable distribution of stem cells to the foot using the cephalic vein approach. Regional limb perfusion through the lateral palmar digital vein with a metacarpal tourniquet were performed. These resulted in the distribution of the stem cells to the foot of all 6 limbs injected, however a marked asymmetry in the distribution was observed, with the radiolabeled stem cells remaining mostly in the area of the lateral palmar digital vein and coronary band vascular plexus.[11] This study confirmed the limitation of the venous regional limb perfusion for proper stem cell distribution and provided reassuring information regarding the safety of the intra-arterial injection technique in the absence of a tourniquet.[11]

All the work described above had been performed under general anesthesia. For broader clinical use it was important to assess these techniques on standing horses. When cephalic vein regional limb perfusion was performed in standing horses, further limitations became apparent.[12] The distal distribution of the radiolabeled was even more limited than when performed under anesthesia, with radioactive signal appreciated distal to the proximal metacarpus in only 3 of 6 limbs (**Fig. 2**A).[12] Furthermore, despite the use of a pneumatic tourniquet, there was evidence of radioactive signal proximal to the tourniquet while it was still in place. Radioactive signal quantification confirmed a much lower retention of stem cells in the distal limb.[12] This difference in efficiency of the tourniquet can be explained by the tension of the forearm muscles that are engaged as the horse is standing, resulting in a less efficient compression of the vessels.

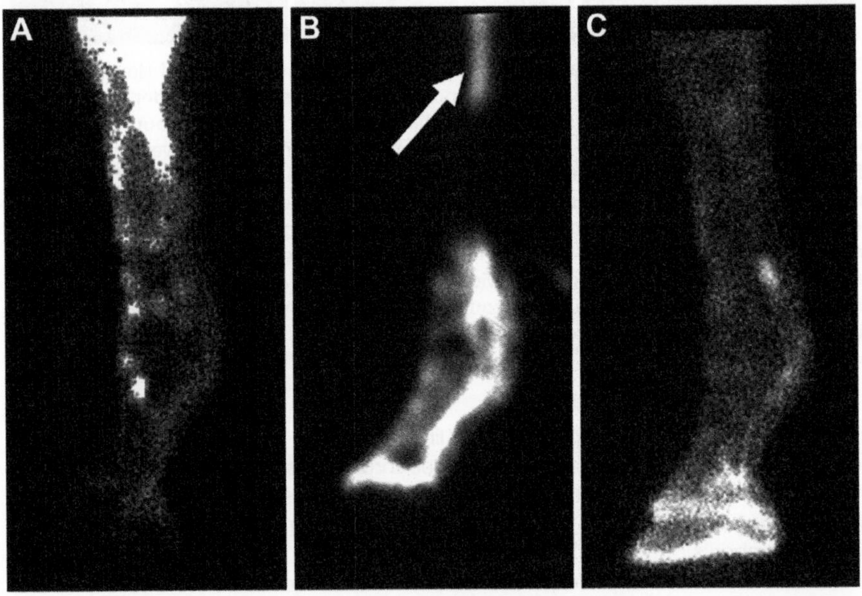

Fig. 2. Lateral scintigraphic images of the distal limb after the injection of HMPAO labeled mesenchymal stem cells in standing horses. (*A*) Regional limb perfusion of the cephalic vein with pneumatic tourniquet on the antebrachium. The distal distribution of stem cells is even further limited when compared with the anesthetized horses (see **Fig. 1**A) with the majority of the stem cells remaining in the larger vessels at the level of the carpus and proximal metacarpus. (*B*) Regional limb perfusion of the lateral palmar digital vein with a pneumatic tourniquet on the metacarpus. There is improved distal distribution when compared with the cephalic regional limb perfusion, however there is no evidence of distribution of radiolabeled stem cells within the hoof. Radioactive signal proximal to the tourniquet (*arrow*) demonstrates partial tourniquet failure with loss of stem cells to the general circulation. (*C*) Injection of the median artery without the use of a tourniquet. There is improved more diffuse and homogenous distribution of the radiolabeled stem cells, in particular with great retention within the hoof.

Regional limb perfusion through the lateral palmar digital vein was also attempted in six horses using standing sedation.[11] A pneumatic tourniquet was also used, inflated at 450 mm Hg, similarly to what had been done under general anesthesia. In half of the horses, very little radioactive signal was present distal to the injection site and radiolabeled cells could be observed in the vein proximal to the tourniquet, confirming tourniquet failure as observed with the cephalic vein injections (**Fig. 2**B).[11] In the three horses with radiolabeled cells observed distally, the majority of the radioactive signal was observed at the coronary band but unlike what had been seen under general anesthesia, very little radioactive signal was seen further distally in the hoof area (see **Fig. 2**B).[11] This was attributed to the difference in pressure within the hoof with the limb being weight-bearing when injection was performed in the standing horses, compared to the non-weight bearing situation in the anesthetized horses.

Catheterizing the median artery in standing horses is more challenging than the cephalic vein due to the deeper location of the artery. Ultrasound is needed for the guidance of the catheter. Another challenge is the risk of arterial spasm that can be triggered while attempting to advance the catheter in the artery. The feasibility of placing median artery catheter was evaluated in 6 research horses.[13] Although all catheter were successfully placed, arterial spasm was identified as a high occurrence. Also, despite the successful placement of the catheter, a horse taking a few steps with the catheter in place was sufficient to induce arterial spasm and retract the catheter out of the artery.[13] For this reason, it was decided that direct needle injection in the median artery with ultrasound guidance should be preferred to catheter placement in standing horses. The main risk with direct needle injection was a risk of partial periarterial injection if motion occurs during the injection.[13] Radiolabeled stem cells were injected using the ultrasound-guided needle injection technique in 6 limbs in research horses.[14] Injections were successful with proper distribution of the radiolabeled stem cells in the distal limb in 5 of the 6 limbs. Strong radioactive signal was present within the hoof, unlike with the palmar digital vein injection in standing horses (**Fig. 2**C). In one limb, although some radiolabeled cells were identified distributing through the distal limb, the majority of the radioactive cells appeared to remain at the injection site, indicating peri-arterial injection of the majority of the cells.[14] There was no evidence of arterial thrombosis in any of these horses.[14]

Based on the advantages of stem cell injection through the median artery when compared with the venous routes, there was a need to develop a technique for intra-arterial injection on the hind limbs. Based on ease of accessibility, the cranial tibial artery at the distal aspect of the tibia was identified as a possible site.[15] Catheterization and angiography were first performed under general anesthesia, confirming the feasibility of the technique. Radiolabeled stem cells were then injected using ultrasound-guided needle injection similarly to what had been performed with the median artery.[15] All 6 injected limbs demonstrated distribution and retention of stem cells in the entire distal limb from distal to the injection site to the foot.[15] The pattern was similar to what was observed in the front limbs with the injection of the median artery.

Further validation of the arterial injection technique was performed using positron emission tomography (PET) for stem cell tracking.[16] Two horses with natural deep digital flexor tendon lesions were injected in the median artery with 18F-Fluorodeoxyglucose labeled stem cells. The PET images confirmed presence of stem cells at the site of tendon lesions (**Fig. 3**).[16]

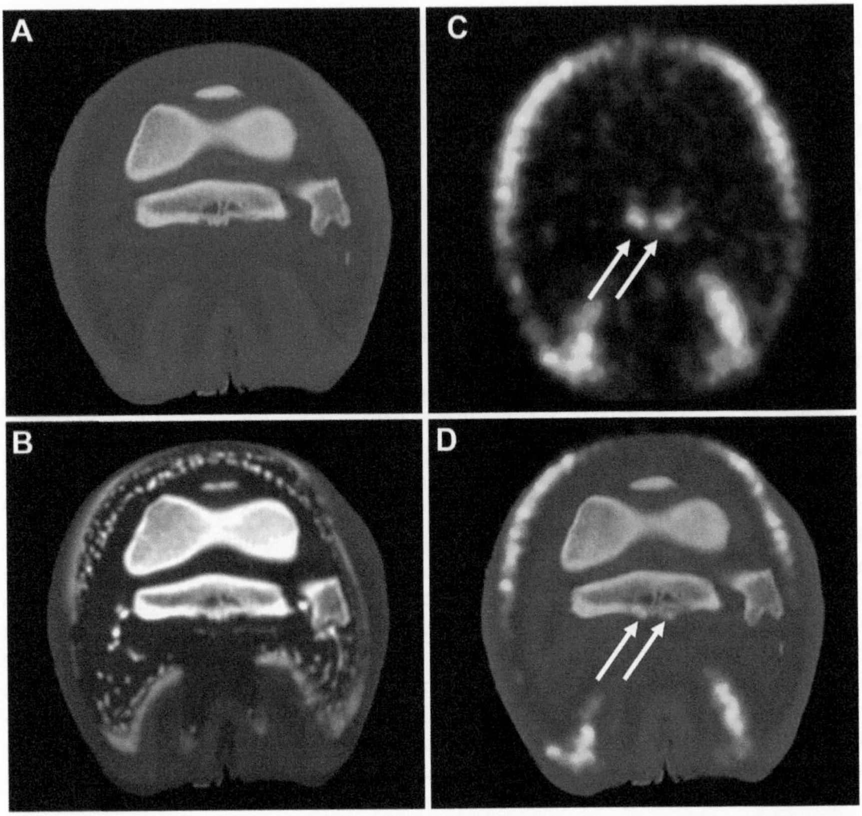

Fig. 3. Computed tomography pre-contrast (*A*) and post arterial contrast (*B*) of the foot of a horse with lysis of the flexor surface of the navicular bone and associated deep digital flexor tendon injury. Positron Emission Tomography (PET) (*C*) and fused PET/CT images (*D*) of the same foot after the injection of the median artery with 18F-Fluorodeoxyglucose (18F-FDG) labeled mesenchymal stem cells. In addition to 18F-FDG labeled stem cell distribution in the highly vascularized coronary band and solar regions, there is focal accumulation of stem cells at the site of navicular bone and deep digital flexor tendon lesions (*arrows*).

Based on these tracking stem cell studies, it was considered that injections of the median artery for the front limb or cranial tibial artery for the hind limb should be the preferred vascular injections techniques for the stem cell treatment of distal limb lesions.

TECHNICAL ASPECTS OF INTRA-ARTERIAL INJECTIONS IN STANDING HORSES

Ultrasound-Guided Injection of the Median Artery

The site for the injection of the median artery is located at the medial aspect of the antebrachium, typically just dorsal and distal to the chestnut.[13,17] A high-frequency linear (8–24 MHz) or mid-frequency (3–11 MHz) microconvex transducer are recommended for guidance. The benefit of the high-frequency linear transducer is maximal resolution. The benefit of the mid-frequency microconvex curvilinear transducer is its small foot print, allowing for greater manipulation of the needle angle and position without the need to adjust the position of the transducer. A subcutaneous line block alone or a median nerve block in combination with a subcutaneous line block proximal to the injection site provides the best regional anesthesia and minimizes the likelihood of arteriospasm. The patient should be sedated sufficiently to remain quiet but not heavily sedated to avoid buckling at the carpus. Additionally, high doses of sedation can cause vasoconstriction, resulting in a more challenging injection. Depending on the patient's temperament, a twitch can also be useful to help maintain a more stationary position. The site should be first be examined with ultrasound and the location for injection determined proximal to the bifurcation of the radial artery prior to preparing the limb. The limb should then prepared aseptically. Two operators are needed for the procedure: one operator aseptically handling the ultrasound probe and the needle, and a second operator, handling the 3-way stop cock and syringes. The operator will be stationed contralateral to the limb being injected in order to readily access the medial aspect of the limb (**Fig. 4**A). The ultrasound machine should be placed to maximize operator comfort. One possibility is to place the machine cranial and lateral to the limb to inject, allowing the operator to face the machine, but bringing the challenge of having the operator and the machine on different sides of the horse. Some operators are more comfortable with placing the machine facing the horse at approximately at the level of the horse's shoulder contralateral to the limb to be injected with the contralateral forelimb placed cranial to the affected limb. A 19 gauge, 3.8 cm needle connected to an extension set flushed with saline solution and connected to a 3-

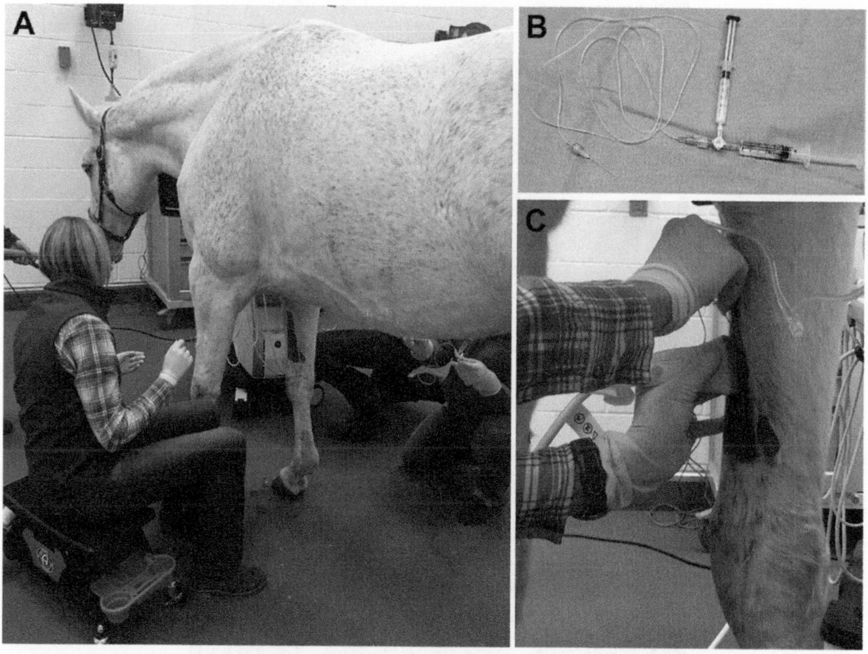

Fig. 4. (*A*) Set-up for the injection of the right median artery of a horse. The injection site, cranial and proximal to the chestnut has been aseptically prepared. The operator is sitting to the left of the horse on a wheel-stool. The ultrasound machine is in front and to the right of the horse. The assistant in charge of operating the syringes is also to the right of the horse. (*B*) Injection set-up consisting of a 19-G needle mounted on a pediatric extension set with a 3-way stop cock with a syringe containing the stem cells and a flush syringe. (*C*) Operator holding probe and needle in place for the injection of the right median artery.

way stop cock with one flush syringe and one syringe loaded with the stem cells should be used (**Fig. 4**B). A pediatric extension set is recommended if available, as it decreases the necessary volume of flush. A longitudinal ultrasound image perfectly centered on the median artery should be obtained. The typical window is located just cranial and proximal to the chestnut (**Fig. 4**C). The median artery is typically identified as a 3 to 8 mm wide vessels deep to the flexor carpi radialis, approximately 10 to 20 mm deep to the skin surface (**Fig. 5**A). The artery can be distinguished from the vein by it visible hypoechoic wall and its pulsatile nature. The vein is readily compressible with probe pressure whereas the artery is not. The preferred injection site is deep

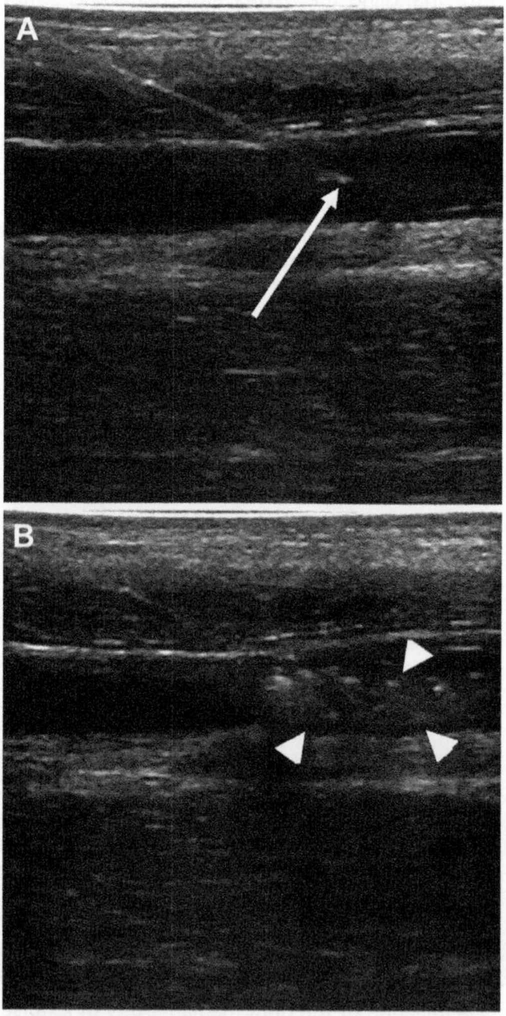

Fig. 5. Ultrasonographic image of a median artery (hypoechoic linear structure) deep to the flexor carpi radialis. (Proximal is to the left) (*A*) A needle is seen inserted proximal to the footprint of the ultrasound transducer and reaching the arterial lumen (*arrow*) (*B*) Same location as image A, obtained while injecting stem cells. The heterogenous echogenic signal (*arrow heads*) demonstrates turbulent flow as the stem cells are successfully injected in the blood stream.

to the distal aspect of the flexor carpi radialis muscle belly, which has a triangular distal contour that helps serve as an imaging landmark. The muscle belly acts as an acoustic stand-off, allowing for proper visualization of the needle position prior to attempting penetrating the wall of the artery.[13] The radial artery can be recognized branching out of the median artery. The preferred injection site is proximal to the radial artery. Once the proper ultrasound image is obtained, the needle is introduced just proximal to the ultrasound probe, in a proximal to distal orientation, approximately 30° to the skin surface (see **Fig. 4**C). The needle should be visualized in the flexor carpi radialis muscle, superficial to the median artery. Care should taken to visualize the tip of the needle at all times because it can be easy to see only a portion of the needle, losing the visualization of the needle tip if the transducer is slightly obliquely oriented. This could lead to inadvertent complete penetration of the needle through the far side of the artery or for the needle to be angled out the plane of the artery. The tip of the needle should be advanced close to the medial wall of the artery, and once the position of the needle is confirmed perfectly aligned with the center of the lumen, the needle is sharply advanced to penetrate through the wall to locate the tip in the center of the lumen (see **Fig. 5**A). The flush syringe is then aspirated to confirm arterial blood can be pulled in the extension set. Once this is confirmed the 3-way stop cock is operated to allow the injection of the stem cells followed by flushing. Typically, successful injections can be appreciated by the visualization of turbulent flow in the lumen of the artery (**Fig. 5**B). In case of periarticular injection, accumulation of hypoechoic fluid and/or gas can be appreciated adjacent to the artery. Real-time ultrasonographic monitoring of the injection is crucial to insure intra-arterial placement throughout the injection. Movements as small as swaying from sedation can alter the position of the needle and necessitate redirection. If there is extravasation of the injectate, the injection should be aborted and the needle replaced at a slightly more distal site. The total injection time is typically limited to 10 to 30 seconds after which the needle is immediately removed and compression using gauze is performed manually for approximately 1 minute, prior to securing the gauze in place with an adhesive elastic band to maintain compression. If there has been any extravasation of the injectate, a full stack wrap is recommended as some horses will develop edema or localized cellulitis.

Ultrasound-Guided Injection of the Cranial Tibial Artery

The same material as described for the median artery injection should be used. The site for the injection of the cranial tibial artery is located at the craniolateral aspect of the distal tibia (**Fig. 6**A).[15] The operator handling the needle and ultrasound probe typically sits on the side of the limb to be injected, cranial and lateral to the limb, with the ultrasound machine positioned caudal and lateral to the limb. A peroneal nerve block and line block or a line block in isolation should be performed prior to injection. The sedation and restraint protocol are similar to the forelimb. At the level of the distal tibia, the cranial tibial artery has a straight course and is relatively superficial, only covered by the thin distal aspect of the long digital extensor muscle. The size of the arterial lumen typically ranges from 2 to 5 mm. Two satellite veins are closely associated with the cranial tibial artery. In some cases, the vein can be congested complicating the access to the artery; however in the authors' experience, there is little complication to penetrating the vein while gaining access to the artery if necessary. It is likely that inactivity contributes to venous congestion. Walking or trotting the horse immediately prior to injection was found helpful to decrease the size of the veins and potentially increase the size of the lumen of the artery. The reference image for injection consists in a longitudinal image of the cranial tibial artery at the distal aspect of the muscle of the long digital extensor (**Fig. 6**B). Similar to the median artery injection, the

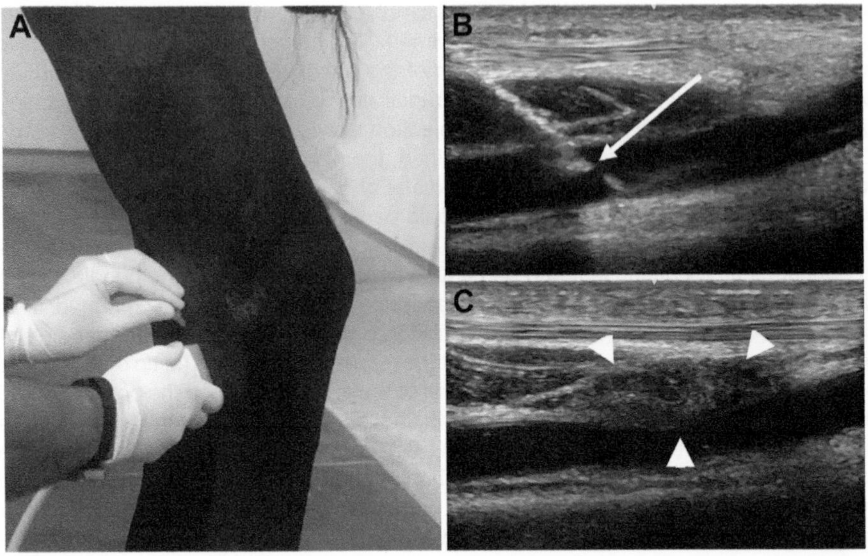

Fig. 6. (*A*) Photograph demonstrating the position of the ultrasound transducer and needle for the injection of the left cranial tibial artery. (*B*) Ultrasonographic image of the cranial tibial artery visualized deep to the long digital extensor muscle, with a needle penetrating into the arterial lumen (*arrow*). The echogenic signal in the artery demonstrates successful injection of stem cells in the lumen. (*C*) Ultrasonographic image obtained at the same site as image B. The heterogenous signal in between the muscle and the artery (*arrowheads*) demonstrates partial peri-arterial injection of the stem cells.

needle is introduced from proximal to the transducer, in a proximal to distal direction at an angle of approximately 30° to the skin surface, using the long digital extensor muscle as a natural stand-off pad to localize the needle prior to artery penetration (see **Fig. 6**A). The artery penetration and injection techniques are similar to the front limb. Successful injection is also confirmed by the visualization of turbulent flow in the artery lumen. In case of periarterial injection, heterogenous hypoechoic material is seen accumulating adjacent to the artery (**Fig. 6**C).

CLINICAL APPLICATIONS

Arterial stem cell injections have been performed in over 100 clinical cases between UC Davis and Colorado State University. These included a majority of autologous bone marrow-derived stem cell injections, but allogenic cells have also been injected intra-arterially. The number of injected cells per limb typically ranged from 10 to 25 million cells, typically suspended in 6 to 10 mL of saline. Most horses at one institution received multiple injections, up to 4 per limb, typically separated by 1 to 2 months. At the other institution, most horses were injected a single time, with less than half receiving additional injections. Injections of the median artery represent the vast majority, but cranial tibial artery injections have been performed in at least 10 horses.

These injections have been used to treat a wide range of injuries. The most common applications have been the treatment of tendon and ligament injuries including the deep digital flexor tendon, the superficial digital flexor tendon, the suspensory ligament, collateral ligaments of the distal interphalangeal joint or distal sesamoidean ligaments. A few osseous lesions such as degenerative changes of the navicular bone or subchondral injuries have also been treated intra-arterially. This technique can be quite useful in horses with navicular apparatus disease that affects both osseous and soft tissue structures. Advanced imaging played an important role in case selection. Visualization of neovascularization or increased blood flow to a lesion using arterial contrast enhanced CT, fluid signal on MRI, doppler ultrasound or increased uptake on positron emission tomography (PET) has been extremely helpful.

A study looking at complications is currently in preparation but overall the rate of complication has been low with less than 10% of horses showing transient mild swelling of the injected limb and very few horses presenting transient increased lameness in the 48 hours following the injection. Non-steroidal anti-inflammatories injection and proper bandaging tends to decrease the risk of complication. In one author's experience, complications are more common in horses undergoing repeat injections.

SUMMARY

Vascular injections of stem cells are a pertinent alternative to direct intralesional injections when treating multiple or extensive lesions or with lesions impossible to reach directly. Extensive research using stem cell tracking has shown that intra-arterial injections without the use of a tourniquet should be preferred over venous or arterial regional limb perfusion techniques using a tourniquet. Proper efficacy studies are still lacking but early clinical work seems promising.

CLINICS CARE POINTS

- Regional vascular injections can be used to administer stem cells to treat musculoskeletal lesions in the equine distal limb.
- Both venous and arterial injection routes have been investigated using stem cell tracking.
- Venous injections require the use of a tourniquet and are limited in term of proper distribution of the stem cells to the distal limb.
- Arterial injection techniques need to be performed without a tourniquet to avoid a potential risk of arterial thrombosis.
- Arterial injection techniques result in better distribution of stem cells to the entire distal limb when compared with venous injection techniques.
- The preferred arterial injection sites are the median artery for the front limbs and the cranial tibial artery for the hind limbs.

REFERENCES

1. Colbath AC, Dow SW, McIlwraith CW, et al. Mesenchymal stem cells for treatment of musculoskeletal disease in horses: Relative merits of allogeneic versus autologous stem cells. Equine Vet J 2020;52:654–63.
2. Schnabel LV, Fortier LA, McIlwraith CW, et al. Therapeutic use of stem cells in horses: which type, how, and when? Vet J 2013;197:570–7.
3. Smith RK, Werling NJ, Dakin SG, et al. Beneficial effects of autologous bone marrow-derived mesenchymal stem cells in naturally occurring tendinopathy. PLoS One 2013;8:e75697.
4. Salz RO, Elliott CRB, Zuffa T, et al. Treatment of racehorse superficial digital flexor tendonitis: A comparison of stem cell treatments to controlled exercise

rehabilitation in 213 cases. Equine Veterinary Journal.n/a 2023. https://doi.org/10.1111/evj.13922.
5. Scharf A, Holmes SP, Thoresen M, et al. MRI-Based Assessment of Intralesional Delivery of Bone Marrow-Derived Mesenchymal Stem Cells in a Model of Equine Tendonitis. Stem Cell Int 2016;2016:8610964.
6. Vallance SA, Vidal MA, Whitcomb MB, et al. Evaluation of a diode laser for use in induction of tendinopathy in the superficial digital flexor tendon of horses. Am J Vet Res 2012;73:1435–44.
7. Becerra P, Valdés Vázquez MA, Dudhia J, et al. Distribution of injected technetium(99m)-labeled mesenchymal stem cells in horses with naturally occurring tendinopathy. J Orthop Res 2013;31:1096–102.
8. Kol A, Walker NJ, Galuppo LD, et al. Autologous point-of-care cellular therapies variably induce equine mesenchymal stem cell migration, proliferation and cytokine expression. Equine Vet J 2013;45:193–8.
9. Sole A, Spriet M, Galuppo LD, et al. Scintigraphic evaluation of intra-arterial and intravenous regional limb perfusion of allogeneic bone marrow-derived mesenchymal stem cells in the normal equine distal limb using (99m) Tc-HMPAO. Equine Vet J 2012;44:594–9.
10. Sole A, Spriet M, Padgett KA, et al. Distribution and persistence of technetium-99 hexamethyl propylene amine oxime-labelled bone marrow-derived mesenchymal stem cells in experimentally induced tendon lesions after intratendinous injection and regional perfusion of the equine distal limb. Equine Vet J 2013;45:726–31.
11. Trela JM, Spriet M, Padgett KA, et al. Scintigraphic comparison of intra-arterial injection and distal intravenous regional limb perfusion for administration of mesenchymal stem cells to the equine foot. Equine Vet J 2014;46:479–83.
12. Spriet M, Buerchler S, Trela JM, et al. Scintigraphic tracking of mesenchymal stem cells after intravenous regional limb perfusion and subcutaneous administration in the standing horse. Vet Surg 2015;44:273–80.
13. Spriet M, Trela JM, Galuppo LD. Ultrasound-guided injection of the median artery in the standing sedated horse. Equine Vet J 2015;47:245–8.
14. Espinosa P, Spriet M, Sole A, et al. Scintigraphic Tracking of Allogeneic Mesenchymal Stem Cells in the Distal Limb After Intra-Arterial Injection in Standing Horses. Vet Surg 2016;45:619–24.
15. Torrent A, Spriet M, Espinosa-Mur P, et al. Ultrasound-guided injection of the cranial tibial artery for stem cell administration in horses. Equine Vet J 2019;51:681–7.
16. Spriet M, Espinosa P, Walker NJ, et al. Preliminary experience with positron emission tomography stem cell tracking in the horse. Sacramento, CA: Proceedings of the the 2018 North American Veterinary Regenerative Medicine Conference; 2018.
17. Barrett M. How To Perform an ultrasound-guided intra-arterial stem cell injections in the median artery. AAEP Proceedings 2019;65:309–13.

Interactions Between Biologic Therapies and Other Treatment Modalities

Aimee C. Colbath, VMD, PhD, DACVS-LA[a,*],
Christopher W. Frye, DVM, DACVSMR[b]

KEYWORDS

- Biologic therapies • Stem cell • Platelet-rich plasma
- Autologous conditioned serum • Laser • Shockwave • Hyperbaric oxygen therapy
- Therapeutic modalities

KEY POINTS

- A horse's health status, exercise, stress, and current medications may affect the quality and efficacy of harvested biologic therapies.
- Pharmaceutical agents (NSAIDs, anxiolytics, and antibiotics), supplements, and therapeutic modalities should be carefully considered when harvesting and administering biologic therapies.
- Laser therapy and extracorporeal shockwave therapy may be combined with biologic therapies, but further research is necessary to understand optimal combination therapy.
- Hyperbaric oxygen therapy may positively affect the quality of harvested biologic therapies and should be further investigated.

INTRODUCTION

Biologic therapies are becoming increasingly popular for the treatment of veterinary species. Recent surveys of large animal practitioners indicate a steady increase in use and many of these therapies are available stall-side from ambulatory veterinarians.[1,2] The veterinary industry has also seen a steady increase in the use of other treatment modalities including physical rehabilitation, specialized shoeing, acupuncture, massage, hydrotherapy, mesotherapy, extracorporeal shockwave, pulsed electromagnetic field therapy (PEMF), chiropractic, laser therapy, and so forth.[3] The growing American College of Sports Medicine and Rehabilitation reflects increasing interest in collaborative and comprehensive treatment and rehabilitation protocols.

[a] Department of Clinical Sciences, Cornell University College of Veterinary Medicine, 930 Campus Road, Box 30, Ithaca, NY 14853, USA; [b] Department of Clinical Sciences, Cornell University College of Veterinary Medicine, 930 Campus Road, Box 25, Ithaca, NY 14853, USA
* Corresponding author.
E-mail address: ac2399@cornell.edu

Vet Clin Equine 39 (2023) 515–523
https://doi.org/10.1016/j.cveq.2023.06.002
vetequine.theclinics.com

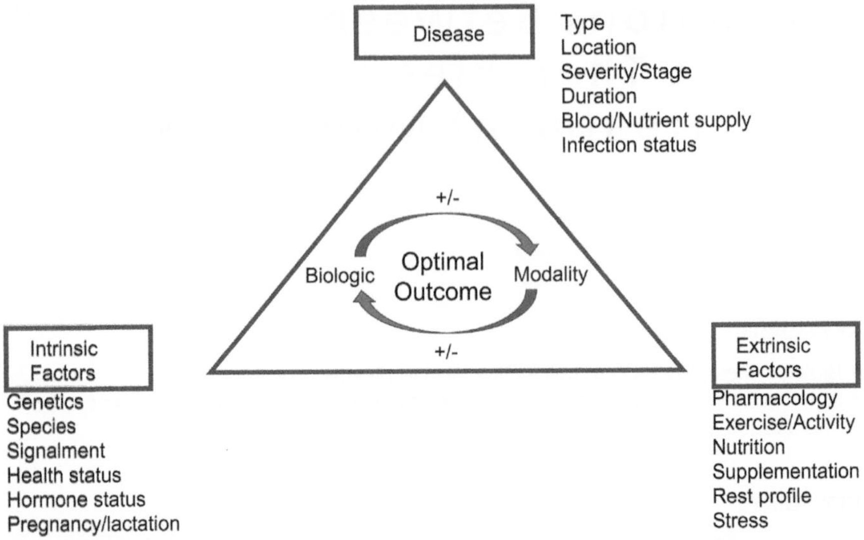

Fig. 1. *Interactions of biologic therapies with other treatment modalities.* The figure illustrates disease considerations, intrinsic factors, and extrinsic factors that must be considered when combining biologic therapies with other treatment modalities.

A recent study investigating the use of therapeutics prior to mesenchymal stromal/stem cell (MSC) therapy for musculoskeletal injury revealed that the use of other therapeutic methods prior to MSC administration resulted in a significantly better outcome than MSC use alone.[4] Likewise, a narrative review of human mechanobiology-based physical therapy modalities performed following orthobiologic administration argues that combining mechanobiologic interventions (taping, bracing, cold immersion, shockwave) with orthobiologics may lead to improved treatment outcomes.[5] This introduces an important concept, that biologic therapies are not given in a vacuum and are often accompanied by other treatment modalities. Furthermore, the optimal application of biologic products depends on a multitude of intrinsic and extrinsic factors including those that may be influenced by therapeutic modalities. Therefore, to utilize biologic therapies most effectively, we must understand their interaction with other treatment types. Owners are increasingly eager to employ multiple treatments and care specialists for the best outcome, and we have a responsibility as treating veterinarians to provide a comprehensive, thoughtful treatment plan for the resolution of the injury (**Fig. 1**).

The literature on the interaction between biologic therapies and other treatment modalities remains in its infancy but is steadily growing. The objective of this article is to review the currently available literature regarding interactions between biologic therapies and other treatment modalities.

DISCUSSION

Biologic Therapies

Multiple biologic therapies are now available in veterinary species. A biologic therapy can be defined as therapy which uses substances from a living organism to treat disease. These may be from the animal itself, defined as autologous, or other animals, defined as allogeneic. According to a recent survey study investigating the use of biologic therapies by large animal specialists, the most used biologic therapy was platelet-rich plasma (PRP) followed by autologous conditioned serum (ACS), bone marrow-derived MSCs (BMDMSCs), autologous protein solution (APS), and adipose-derived MSCs (ADMSCs).[1] Other biologic therapies available to veterinary practitioners include platelet lysate, alpha-2 macroglobulin, and placentally derived products such as liquid amnion allograph. Products such as alpha-2 macroglobulin and liquid amnion allograph have limited equine studies to date.[6]

Health and Age

For autologous biologic therapies, consideration needs to be given to the health status of the individual. Animal health, age, and other interventions (pharmaceutical administration, exercise, stress, and so forth) may affect the characteristics of the biologic therapy, further warranting the exploration of physical and pharmaceutical interventions with biologic therapies. In contrast, allogeneic therapies may have the ability to be more consistent and controlled. However, the concern for potential adverse immune-mediated reactions must be considered in addition to the influence of other treatment modalities.[7]

In horses, donor age has been linked with a reduction in chondrogenic and osteogenic differentiation of both BMDMSCs and ADMSCs.[8] Likewise, in humans and mouse experiments chondrocytes treated with PRP from young donors resulted in a more "youthful" chondrocyte phenotype and improved cartilage health in comparison to PRP from older individuals.[9]

Studies identifying variables which may optimize biologic therapies are necessary. For example, PRP concentration and cellular content in horses were associated with the time of blood draw, hydration status, anti-inflammatory drug use, and training periods. The study indicated that horses receiving ketoprofen, a non-steroidal anti-inflammatory, had a higher platelet concentration while horses exposed to exercise and dehydration had a higher white blood cell count within harvested PRP.[10] However, platelet count should not be mistaken as a measure of PRP efficacy. Optimization of PRP therapy includes understanding the effects of platelet count, associated growth factor release, and influence of the white blood cell profile. An additional study has suggested that factors such as horse breed, gender, and age may influence levels of growth factors such as platelet-derived growth factor – BB concentrations in platelet-rich plasma.[11] Optimizing such effects may be further complicated by the signalment, health, anatomic site of administration, method of administration, dosing, and stage of the disease. With many potential variables affecting the quality of PRP and its healing potential, there are significant research opportunities for optimizing this therapy where multiple variables should be considered.

Exercise and Stress

Recent exercise or bouts of stress may also lead to alterations in biologic therapies. For example, a single bout of intense exercise resulted in reduced interleukin-1 receptor antagonist (IL-1Ra) concentrations in ACS compared to horses at rest, suggesting that ACS should not be harvested within 24 hours of intense exercise.[12] This is particularly important as an in vivo study in harness horses suggests that the therapeutic benefits of ACS may be linked to the concentration of IL-1Ra and IGF-1 within the ACS administered.[13] For convenience, some clinicians may want to harvest ACS following a surgical procedure such as arthroscopy or tenoscopy for future treatment. Unfortunately, similar to intense exercise, surgical stress may also lead to significant changes in ACS cytokine profiles with one study suggesting that ACS samples from horses with marked surgical stress have lower concentrations of IL-1Ra compared to samples harvested from the same animal prior to surgical stress.[14] These findings suggest that, if possible, ACS should be harvested before surgery or potentially prior to hospital admission.

Concurrent Pharmaceutical Administration

Horses receiving biologic therapies may be receiving pharmaceutical interventions such as non-steroidal anti-inflammatories (NSAIDs) or calming agents. These medications may have a significant effect on the composition or quality of the biologic therapy. For example, Gilbertie and colleagues (2019) showed reserpine, a commonly utilized long-term tranquilizer with a prolonged half-life in horses, results in significant changes in platelet function including increased aggregation and adhesion resulting in hypercoagulability and suggesting PRP should be harvested prior to reserpine use.[15] Likewise, the administration of omega-3 and omega-6 fatty acids in cats resulted in decreased platelet aggregation and altered platelet function.[16] Further, NSAIDs have been found to exert effects on the proliferation, migration, and differentiation of MSCs with a dose-dependent effect. At lower concentrations NSAIDs may promote proliferation, while at higher concentrations they may decrease proliferation and inhibit osteogenic differentiation.[17] In contrast, a recent study by Ludwig and colleagues (2017) found NSAIDs did not influence platelet activation, growth factor release or TXB2 production with HGT as an activator in canine platelet-rich plasma.[18] These studies highlight an important point to practitioners that harvest biologic therapies. Namely, other pharmaceutical interventions may affect the composition and potentially the efficacy of biologic therapies and response could vary between species. Therefore, concurrent administration of other pharmaceuticals should be further researched and carefully considered.

Biologic therapies may also be strategically combined with other pharmaceuticals. For example, MSCs have antibacterial effects,[19] and may be strategically combined with antibiotic therapies to target difficult bacterial infections. However, concurrent local administration of some antibiotics (depending on the dose) and MSCs should be avoided. For example, equine BMDMSCs incubated with gentamicin and amikacin resulted in the death of greater than 95% of MSCs in less than 2 hours.[20] In addition, MSCs exposed to enrofloxacin and ceftiofur had decreased cell viability in vitro.[21] Platelet lysate also has documented antibacterial effects and may be a particularly valuable treatment for synovial sepsis and biofilm formation.[22–24] In an in vivo experimental study of synovial sepsis, the combination of amikacin with a platelet lysate product resulted in a reduced bacterial concentration and as well as decreased inflammation and fibrosis.[22] Platelet lysate, as a non-cellular therapy, may be concurrently administered with antibiotics without concern of cellular viability.

It is also important to realize that systemic pharmaceuticals may be present within the biologic therapy harvested. For example, an equine study showed the administration of firocoxib systemically led to detectable levels of firocoxib within harvested autologous conditioned serum.[25] Although levels were not high enough to elicit a positive plasma drug test following intra-articular administration, it is important to realize a systemic drug may be inadvertently administered locally (ex. intra-articularly) due to its presence within a biologic therapeutic. This may be especially important to avoid for cartilage toxic drugs such as some systemic antibiotics that may be administered peri-operatively.[26–28]

Extracorporeal Shockwave Therapy

Non-pharmaceutical interventions such as extracorporeal shockwave therapy or laser therapy may be used in conjunction with biologic therapies. Extracorporeal shockwave therapy is a popular intervention for musculoskeletal disease including desmitis and tendonitis as well as muscle pain.[29] In addition, the therapy has been used in humans to encourage bone healing and treatment of hypertrophic boney non-union.[30] PRP exposed to extracorporeal shockwave in vitro resulted in significant increases in TGF- β_1 and PDGF- $\beta\beta$ compared to the resting PRP sample. Although an in vitro study, the study suggests that combining PRP injection with shockwave application may be beneficial for growth factor release.[31]

In an in vitro study by Colbath and colleagues (2020), extracorporeal shockwave had no negative effects on MSC viability or proliferation and a significant but transient increase in alkaline phosphatase was noted, suggesting extracorporeal shockwave may be safe to perform with MSC injection and further research on osteogenic effects may be warranted in the horse.[32] Raabe and colleagues (2013) demonstrated exposure of ADMSCs to focal shockwave could improve cellular proliferation in vitro without altering differentiation; however, a dose and impulse dependent cytotoxicity was also observed.[33]

The effects of extracorporeal shockwave administered concurrently with ACS and APS in the horse are not well documented. One might expect extracorporeal shockwave to have a lesser effect on these non-cellular therapies. However, research is still warranted especially regarding its effect on tissues at the site of biologic therapy administration.

Laser Therapy

Therapeutic laser also known as photobiomodulation has become a popular ancillary modality for various musculoskeletal and wound healing applications. As a non-invasive therapy it is often combined with other treatment modalities for its perceived pain relieving, anti-inflammatory and pro-healing effects. An in vitro study in horses suggests that photobiomodulation using low-level laser therapy (LLLT) does not result in significant negative effects on BMDMSCs.[34] Further, the study noted an increase in the anti-inflammatory cytokine interleukin-10 and vascular endothelial growth factor when BMDMSCs were exposed to photobiomodulation suggesting LLLT may enhance the anti-inflammatory effects of BMDMSCs.[34] Laser therapy may also influence the differentiation of cells. LLLT in an in vitro study induced a significant increase in tenascin C levels in cultured MSCs, influencing their ability to differentiate into tenocytes.[35] Although significant additional research studies are necessary, this loosely suggests a potential advantage to combining therapeutic laser and MSC administration in tendon injury.

In a surgically induced rabbit and rodent model tendon injury, Achilles tendon healing speed was more efficient when using a combination of LLLT and PRP when compared to control animals.[36,37] The combination therapy is more researched in human skin conditions with the successful treatment of skin scarring and vitiligo (loss of skin color).[38,39] Further, the combination of PRP and laser therapy has shown promise for the resolution of skin infections in animal pre-clinical wound models of MRSA.[40] With the popularity of therapeutic laser increasing especially in combination with other biologic therapies a further understanding of its influence on the tissue environment and biologic therapies is necessary.

In addition to LLLT, high-intensity laser treatment (HILT) has recently gained popularity as a regenerative treatment for tendonitis and desmitis in the horse. HILT uses a class 4 laser that can deliver more energy than the typical LLLT in a shorter duration. A recent experimental study of suspensory branch injury suggests HILT improves lesion healing over conservative management.[41] Further, a case series of horses suffering from lower hock joint arthritis treated solely with HILT, suggested a potential pain-relieving effect of HILT.[42] Although limited studies are currently available in the veterinary literature, this therapy is being used for musculoskeletal conditions commonly treated with biologic therapies. Therefore, additional research is warranted to understand its interaction with biologic therapies.

Hyperbaric Oxygen Therapy

Hyperbaric oxygen therapy has been used in the treatment of gastrointestinal disease, musculoskeletal disease, neurologic disease, respiratory disease, and neonatal asphyxia in the horse.[43] The horse is placed in a sealed chamber and exposed to oxygen that is several times higher than normal atmospheric pressure to forcibly increase oxygen in body fluids and bodily tissues. A study has suggested that exposure of horses to hyperbaric oxygen therapy prior to blood harvest may increase the CD90+ cells in peripheral blood and lead to better proliferative capacity of blood-derived mesenchymal stem cells.[44] However, it is currently unknown how hyperbaric oxygen may affect the secretion of growth factors or paracrine activity of MSCs or its effect on bone marrow-derived or adipose-derived MSCs. Likewise, the effect of hyperbaric oxygen on equine platelet-rich plasma or other biologic therapies is currently unknown. That stated, an in vitro study which exposed equine platelets to hyperbaric oxygen conditions found no detrimental effects on platelet biochemistry and no evidence of oxidative stress.[45] Hyperbaric oxygen therapy has the potential to significantly effect biologic therapies as well as the tissue receiving biologic therapies, and therefore, an increased understanding of its effects in horses is warranted.

SUMMARY

The demands for comprehensive and multi-modal therapies including the use of both biologic and ancillary treatment modalities continue to rise. Further research is necessary to explore the interactions between biological and ancillary therapies as an important component toward optimizing treatment. Likewise, clinicians employing biological therapies must account for the health status of their patient as well as administered pharmaceuticals, supplements, or modalities.

DISCLOSURE

The authors have nothing to disclose.

CLINICS CARE POINTS

- A horse's health status, exercise, stress, and current medications should be assessed prior to harvesting biologic therapies.
- Ideally biologic therapies should be harvested prior to the administration of other pharmaceutical agents.
- Laser therapy and extracorporeal shockwave therapy may be combined with biologic therapies, but further research is necessary to understand optimal combination therapy.
- Hyperbaric oxygen therapy may positively affect the quality of some biologic therapies and should be further investigated.

REFERENCES

1. Knott LE, Fonseca-Martinez BA, O'Connor AM, et al. Current use of biologic therapies for musculoskeletal disease: A survey of board-certified equine specialists. Vet Surg 2022;51:557–67.

2. Velloso Alvarez A, Boone LH, Braim AP, et al. A Survey of Clinical Usage of Non-steroidal Intra-Articular Therapeutics by Equine Practitioners. Front Vet Sci 2020; 7:579967.
3. Wilson JM, McKenzie E, Duesterdieck-Zellmer K. International Survey Regarding the Use of Rehabilitation Modalities in Horses. Front Vet Sci 2018;5:120.
4. Bernardino PN, Smith WA, Galuppo LD, et al. Therapeutics prior to mesenchymal stromal cell therapy improves outcome in equine orthopedic injuries. Am J Vet Res 2022;83. ajvr.22.04.0072.
5. McKay J, Nasb M, Hafsi K. Mechanobiology-based physical therapy and rehabilitation after orthobiologic interventions: a narrative review. Int Orthop 2022;46: 179–88.
6. Duddy HR, Schoonover MJ, Hague BA. Outcome following local injection of a liquid amnion allograft for treatment of equine tendonitis or desmitis – 100 cases. BMC Vet Res 2022;18:391–401.
7. Rowland AL, Miller D, Berglund A, et al. Cross-matching of allogeneic mesenchymal stromal cells eliminates recipient immune targeting. Stem Cells Transl Med 2021;10:694–710.
8. Bagge J, Berg LC, Janes J, et al. Donor age effects on in vitro chondrogenic and osteogenic differentiation performance of equine bone marrow- and adipose tissue-derived mesenchymal stromal cells. BMC Vet Res 2022;18:388.
9. Chowdhary K, Sahu A, Iijima H, et al. Aging Affects the Efficacy of Platelet-Rich Plasma Treatment for Osteoarthritis. Am J Phys Med Rehabil 2022. https://doi.org/10.1097/PHM.0000000000002161.
10. Rinnovati R, Romagnoli N, Gentilini F, et al. The influence of environmental variables on platelet concentration in horse platelet-rich plasma. Acta Vet Scand 2016;58:45.
11. Giraldo CE, Lopez C, Alvarez ME, et al. Effects of the breed, sex and age on cellular content and growth factor release from equine pure-platelet rich plasma and pure-platelet rich gel. BMC Vet Res 2013;9:29.
12. Hale JN, Hughes KJ, Hall S, et al. The effect of exercise on cytokine concentration in equine autologous conditioned serum. Equine Vet J 2022;55(3):551–6.
13. Marques-Smith P, Kallerud AS, Johansen GM, et al. Is clinical effect of autologous conditioned serum in spontaneously occurring equine articular lameness related to ACS cytokine profile? BMC Vet Res 2020;16:181.
14. Fjordbakk CT, Johansen GM, Lovas AC, et al. Surgical stress influences cytokine content in autologous conditioned serum. Equine Vet J 2015;47:212–7.
15. Gilbertie JM, Davis JL, Davidson GS, et al. Oral reserpine administration in horses results in low plasma concentrations that alter platelet biology. Equine Vet J 2019; 51:537–43.
16. Saker KE, Eddy AL, Thatcher CD, et al. Manipulation of dietary (n-6) and (n-3) fatty acids alters platelet function in cats. J Nutr 1998;128:2645S–7S.
17. Muller M, Raabe O, Addicks K, et al. Effects of non-steroidal anti-inflammatory drugs on proliferation, differentiation and migration in equine mesenchymal stem cells. Cell Biol Int 2011;35:235–48.
18. Ludwig HC, Birdwhistell KE, Brainard BM, et al. Use of a Cyclooxygenase-2 Inhibitor Does Not Inhibit Platelet Activation or Growth Factor Release From Platelet-Rich Plasma. Am J Sports Med 2017;45:3351–7.
19. Pezzanite LM, Chow L, Johnson V, et al. Toll-like receptor activation of equine mesenchymal stromal cells to enhance antibacterial activity and immunomodulatory cytokine secretion. Vet Surg 2021;50:858–71.

20. Bohannon LK, Owens SD, Walker NJ, et al. The effects of therapeutic concentrations of gentamicin, amikacin and hyaluronic acid on cultured bone marrow-derived equine mesenchymal stem cells. Equine Vet J 2013;45:732–6.
21. Parker RA, Clegg PD, Taylor SE. The in vitro effects of antibiotics on cell viability and gene expression of equine bone marrow-derived mesenchymal stromal cells. Equine Vet J 2012;44:355–60.
22. Gilbertie JM, Schaer TP, Engiles JB, et al. A Platelet-Rich Plasma-Derived Biologic Clears Staphylococcus aureus Biofilms While Mitigating Cartilage Degeneration and Joint Inflammation in a Clinically Relevant Large Animal Infectious Arthritis Model. Front Cell Infect Microbiol 2022;12:895022.
23. Gilbertie JM, Schaer TP, Schubert AG, et al. Platelet-rich plasma lysate displays antibiofilm properties and restores antimicrobial activity against synovial fluid biofilms in vitro. J Orthop Res 2020;38:1365–74.
24. Gordon J, Alvarez-Narvaez S, Peroni JF. Antimicrobial Effects of Equine Platelet Lysate. Front Vet Sci 2021;8:703414.
25. Ortved KF, Goodale MB, Ober C, et al. Plasma firocoxib concentrations after intra-articular injection of autologous conditioned serum prepared from firocoxib positive horses. Vet J 2017;230:20–3.
26. Newman RJ, Chow L, Goodrich LR, et al. Susceptibility of canine chondrocytes and synoviocytes to antibiotic cytotoxicity in vitro. Vet Surg 2021;50:650–8.
27. Pezzanite L, Chow L, Hendrickson D, et al. Evaluation of Intra-Articular Amikacin Administration in an Equine Non-inflammatory Joint Model to Identify Effective Bactericidal Concentrations While Minimizing Cytotoxicity. Front Vet Sci 2021;8:676774.
28. Pezzanite L, Chow L, Soontararak S, et al. Amikacin induces rapid dose-dependent apoptotic cell death in equine chondrocytes and synovial cells in vitro. Equine Vet J 2020;52:715–24.
29. Bostrom A, Asplund K, Bergh A, et al. Systematic Review of Complementary and Alternative Veterinary Medicine in Sport and Companion Animals: Therapeutic Ultrasound. Animals (Basel) 2022;12:3144.
30. Mittermayr R, Haffner N, Feichtinger X, et al. The role of shockwaves in the enhancement of bone repair - from basic principles to clinical application. Injury 2021;52(Suppl 2):S84–90.
31. Seabaugh KA, Thoresen M, Giguere S. Extracorporeal Shockwave Therapy Increases Growth Factor Release from Equine Platelet-Rich Plasma In Vitro. Front Vet Sci 2017;4:205.
32. Colbath AC, Kisiday JD, Phillips JN, et al. Can Extracorporeal Shockwave Promote Osteogenesis of Equine Bone Marrow-Derived Mesenchymal Stem Cells In Vitro? Stem Cells Dev 2020;29:110–8.
33. Raabe O, Shell K, Goessl A, et al. Effect of extracorporeal shock wave on proliferation and differentiation of equine adipose tissue-derived mesenchymal stem cells in vitro. Am J Stem Cells 2013;2:62–73.
34. Peat FJ, Colbath AC, Bentsen LM, et al. In Vitro Effects of High-Intensity Laser Photobiomodulation on Equine Bone Marrow-Derived Mesenchymal Stem Cell Viability and Cytokine Expression. Photomed Laser Surg 2018;36:83–91.
35. Gomiero C, Bertolutti G, Martinello T, et al. Tenogenic induction of equine mesenchymal stem cells by means of growth factors and low-level laser technology. Vet Res Commun 2016;40:39–48.
36. Allahverdi A, Sharifi D, Takhtfooladi MA, et al. Evaluation of low-level laser therapy, platelet-rich plasma, and their combination on the healing of Achilles tendon in rabbits. Lasers Med Sci 2015;30:1305–13.

37. Barbosa D, de Souza RA, de Carvalho WR, et al. Low-level laser therapy combined with platelet-rich plasma on the healing calcaneal tendon: a histological study in a rat model. Lasers Med Sci 2013;28:1489–94.
38. Chen J, Yu N, Li H, et al. Meta-analysis of the efficacy of adding platelet-rich plasma to 308-nm excimer laser for patients with vitiligo. J Int Med Res 2022; 50. 3000605221119646.
39. Nita AC, Orzan OA, Filipescu M, et al. Fat graft, laser CO(2) and platelet-rich-plasma synergy in scars treatment. J Med Life 2013;6:430–3.
40. Lee WR, Hsiao CY, Huang TH, et al. Low-fluence laser-facilitated platelet-rich plasma permeation for treating MRSA-infected wound and photoaging of the skin. Int J Pharm 2021;595:120242.
41. Pluim M, Heier A, Plomp S, et al. Histological tissue healing following high-power laser treatment in a model of suspensory ligament branch injury. Equine Vet J 2022;54:1114–22.
42. Zielinska P, Sniegucka K, Kielbowicz Z. A Case Series of 11 Horses Diagnosed with Bone Spavin Treated with High Intensity Laser Therapy (HILT). J Equine Vet Sci 2022;120:104188.
43. Geiser DR. Hyperbaric Oxygen Therapy in Equine Rehabilitation: Putting the Pressure on Disease. Vet Clin North Am Equine Pract 2016;32:149–57.
44. Dhar M, Neilsen N, Beatty K, et al. Equine peripheral blood-derived mesenchymal stem cells: isolation, identification, trilineage differentiation and effect of hyperbaric oxygen treatment. Equine Vet J 2012;44:600–5.
45. Shaw FL, Handy RD, Bryson P, et al. A single exposure to hyperbaric oxygen does not cause oxidative stress in isolated platelets: no effect on superoxide dismutase, catalase, or cellular ATP. Clin Biochem 2005;38:722–6.

Use of Biologics and Stem Cells for Wound Healing in the Horse

Rebecca M. Harman, PhD, Aarthi Rajesh, PhD,
Gerlinde R. Van de Walle, DVM, PhD*

KEYWORDS

• Wound healing • Horse • Biologics • Stem cells • Platelet-rich plasma

KEY POINTS

- Biologic therapies, including stem cells and platelet-rich plasma (PRP), have the potential to improve equine skin wound healing based on in vitro data and small in vivo trials.
- Well-controlled clinical studies involving large number of horses are warranted to determine the efficacy of biologic therapies in promoting equine skin wound healing.
- Biologic therapies can be optimized to improve efficacy of equine skin wound healing.

BACKGROUND

Relevance

The diversity of cells that make up the multilayered skin, the largest organ, function together to support homeostasis.[1] The outer epidermis, composed of keratinized, stratified squamous epithelium, provides a protective barrier against pollutants and pathogens and prevents dehydration. The underlying dermis contains nerve endings that receive signals from the environment, glands that produce oils and sweat, and immune cells that serve as the first line of defense against penetrating microbes and toxins. The deepest layer of the skin, the hypodermis, is well-vascularized and consists of abundant adipose tissue to control body temperature. It connects the dermis to muscle and bone to maintain structural integrity (**Fig. 1**). Healthy, uncompromised skin is required for the well-being of horses, making the treatment of skin wounds a high priority in equine medicine.

Processes of Skin Wound Healing

The process of skin wound repair has conventionally been divided into 4 sequential and overlapping stages: hemostasis, inflammation, proliferation, and remodeling

Baker Institute for Animal Health, College of Veterinary Medicine, Cornell University, Ithaca, NY 14853, USA
* Corresponding author.
E-mail address: grv23@cornell.edu

Vet Clin Equine 39 (2023) 525–539
https://doi.org/10.1016/j.cveq.2023.06.003
vetequine.theclinics.com

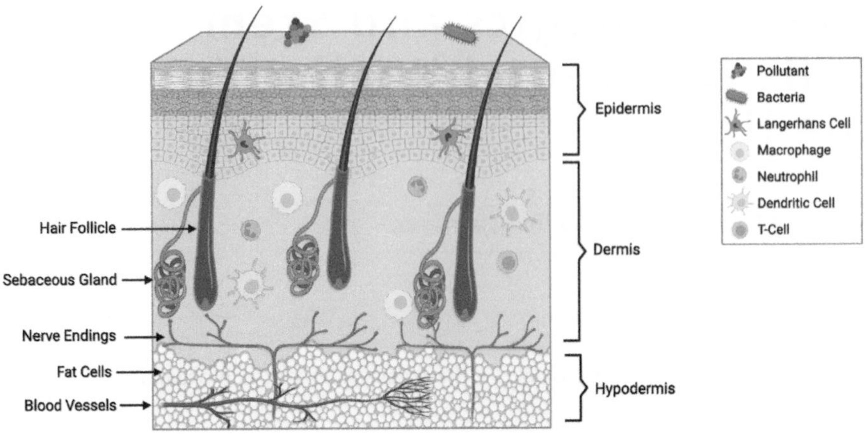

Fig. 1. Skin consists of 3 main layers. The epidermis, which serves as a barrier against pathogens and pollutants and prevents dehydration; the dermis, containing nerve endings, sweat and oil glands and immune cells; and the hypodermis containing blood vessels and fat cells.

(**Fig. 2**). Although these stages are often presented in simple terms, successful healing of full-thickness skin wounds is an intricate process depending on the synchronized interactions of many cell types functioning together to restore skin integrity (**Fig. 3**).[2,3]

Skin Wound Healing Considerations Specific to the Horse

The horse is a unique species with behavioral tendencies and physiological features that affect skin wound formation and healing. Horses are large animals with a "fight or flight" instinct, often living in environments that make them prone to lacerations. Physiologically, the quality and thickness of skin varies across the horse's body.[4] Horses are often described as "tight skinned," like humans, with the skin firmly attached to the underlying connective tissue. However, the skin on their trunk can be categorized as "loose," which is more typical of laboratory rodents.[5] These differences in skin quality correspond to the distribution of the *panniculus carnosus,* a layer of striated muscle beneath the dermis, which stretches from the knees to the base of the neck (**Fig. 4**),[6] and also determine the way in which equine wounds heal. Wounds

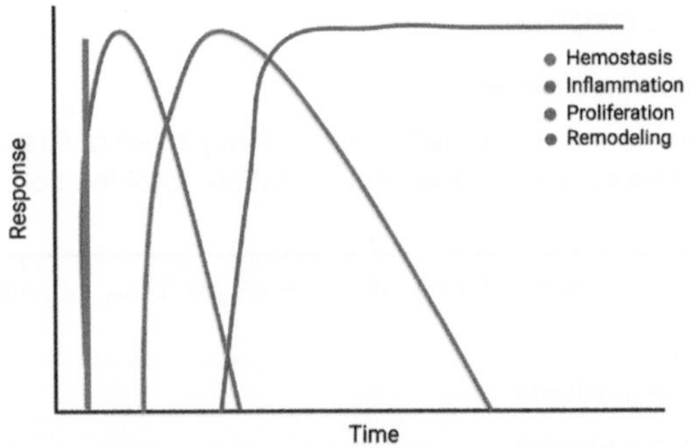

Fig. 2. Skin wound healing is often simply described as occurring in 4 overlapping phases consisting of hemostasis, inflammation, proliferation, and remodeling.

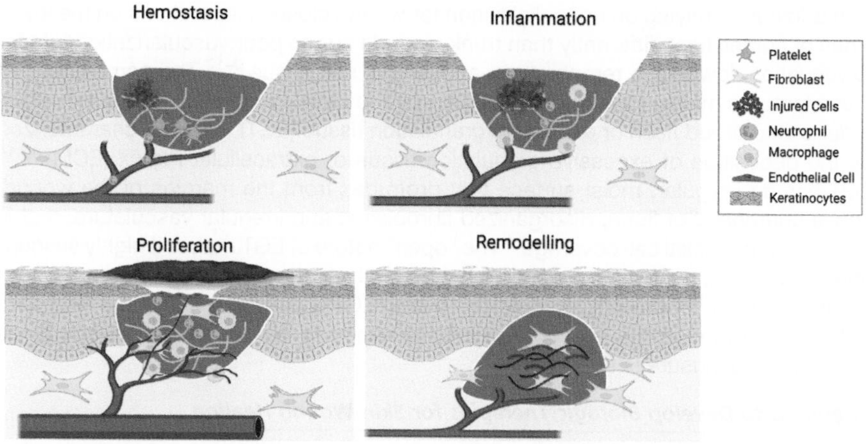

Fig. 3. The 4 phases of skin wound healing involve a complex network of events mediated by various cell types in the skin. During hemostasis, platelets secrete platelet-derived growth factor (PDGF) and transforming growth factor beta (TGFβ) that attract neutrophils and macrophages to the site of injury. During the inflammatory phase, neutrophils secrete TGFβ, while macrophage-derived vascular endothelial growth factor (VEGF), endothelial growth factor (EGF), interleukin-2 (IL-1), tumor necrosis factor alpha (TNFα), and transforming growth factor alpha (TGFα) signal to endothelial cells and keratinocytes in order to initiate angiogenesis and keratinocyte migration in the proliferation phase. During the proliferation phase, endothelial cells secrete fibroblast growth factors (FGFs) and TGFβ, while keratinocytes secrete TGFβ, VEGF, FGFs, and IL-1, which are involved in fibroblast recruitment. During the remodeling phase, fibroblasts secrete FGFs, insulin-like growth factors (IGFs), interferons (IFNs), TGFβ, VEGF, and extracellular matrix (ECM) components, which interact to restore skin integrity.

on the trunk heal similarly to wounds of laboratory rodents, namely by contraction of the *panniculus carnosus*,[7] while distal limb wounds heal like human wounds, with epithelialization of the primary surface, followed by stromal granulation and myofibroblast migration and contraction.[8]

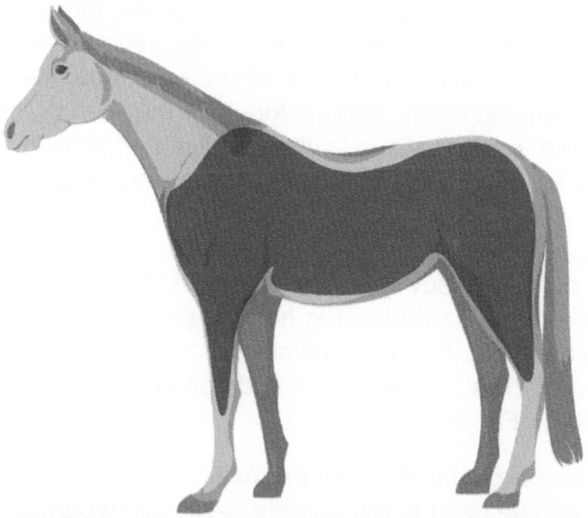

Fig. 4. Distribution of the *panniculus carnosus* muscle in the horse.

In addition to relying on epithelialization for wound closure, lacerations on the lower limbs of horses heal differently than trunk wounds due to poor vascularization/inferior oxygenation, low tissue temperature, and lack of soft tissue.[9–12] The combination of these features makes lower limb wounds prone to developing a fibroproliferative disorder called proud flesh or exuberant granulation tissue (EGT), which is characterized by the deposition of excessive granulation tissue or extracellular matrix (ECM).[13,14] EGT has an irregular, moist surface that protrudes from the margins of the wound, and is composed of fibrin, disorganized fibroblasts, and irregular vasculature, that is resistant to epithelial cell coverage.[4] The "open" nature of EGT makes it highly susceptible to abrasion, reinjury, and secondary bacterial infections, leading to chronic, nonhealing wounds.[15] Currently, surgical removal of EGT is considered the best treatment option, even though the procedure typically needs to be performed several times before wound closure is successful.[13]

Incentives to Develop Biologic Therapies for Skin Wound Healing

Cell-based therapies, including biologic dressings, stem cells and stem cell secreted products, and platelet-rich plasma (PRP), all have the potential to improve skin wound healing nonsurgically by introducing growth factors and cytokines that encourage deposition of healthy ECM molecules, fibroblast migration, angiogenesis, and epithelial cell migration. They also have inherent antimicrobial properties that can discourage bacterial growth, thus reducing the need for conventional antibiotics. Minimizing the use of antibiotics fits within the emerging perspectives on antimicrobial use and stewardship in equine practice[16] and is desirable in light of the global threat of antibiotic-resistant bacteria.[17] Bacteria possess mutation mechanisms, allowing them to adapt rapidly to changes in the environment, including exposure to antibiotics. The misuse and overuse of conventional antibiotics push some bacteria to mutate, survive treatment, and contribute to resistant populations.[18] The multifaceted mechanisms by which biologic therapies can control bacteria in skin wounds may be less likely to lead to resistance than conventional antibiotics.[19]

EVIDENCE FOR THE EFFICACY OF BIOLOGIC THERAPIES FOR EQUINE SKIN WOUNDS

In Vitro Research

The rationale for carrying out in vitro experiments is that understanding how cellular therapies work allows for their refinement in order to improve patient outcomes. To date, these in vitro studies have primarily focused on the bioactive factors secreted by mesenchymal stromal cells (MSCs), called the secretome. Specifically, these studies were designed to define the nature of secreted bioactive factors, determine how they affect resident skin cells, and explore how they can be effectively delivered to wounds.[20–27] **Table 1** summarizes in vitro studies that provide evidence that biologic therapies may be effective at improving the healing of equine skin wounds.

In Vivo Studies

The true measures of the efficacy of biologic therapies for equine skin wounds can be obtained from in vivo work carried out in horses, such as experimentally controlled studies and/or clinical trials. Biologic dressings, stem cells, and PRP have all been tested in small in vivo trials, as described in detail in the following sections and as shown schematically in **Fig. 5**.

Biologic dressings and acellular dressing products

Biologic dressings can be used to temporarily cover skin wounds, provide protection of healing tissues, serve as a barrier to microbes, and promote wound maturation.[28]

Table 1
Summary of *in vitro* studies of cell-based therapies for equine skin wounds

Cell and/or Cell Product	Main Findings/Conclusions
Equine PB-MSC secretome	Promotes equine EC proliferation and endothelial tube-like formation. Endothelin-1, IGFBP-2, IL-8, and PDGF-AA are present in PB-MSC secretome and induce the expression of VEGF-A on EC, leading to endothelial tube-like formation. → PB-MSC secretome may promote angiogenesis in vivo.
Equine PB-MSC secretome, PB-MSCs	PB-MSC secretome promotes equine DF migration. PB-MSCs encapsulated in double-layer microparticles remain viable, retain stem cell characteristics, and secrete factors that promote DF migration. → Encapsulated PB-MSC may improve wound healing in vivo.
Equine PB-MSC secretome	PB-MSC secretome blocks TGF-β1–induced changes in equine DF morphology and function. PB-MSC CM also alters the phenotype of DF isolated from equine EGT. → PB-MSC secretome has the potential to reduce EGT in vivo.
Equine PB-MSC secretome	PB-MSC secretome inhibits the growth of *E coli* and *S aureus* and secretes AMPs. Blocking AMP activity in the secretome reduces secretome effects on bacteria. → PB-MSC secretome may inhibit bacterial growth in equine skin wounds.
Equine PB-MSC secretome	PB-MSC secretome contains PAI-1 and tenascin-C that promote DF migration, decrease DF adhesion, and reduce anisotropy of actin in DFs. These factors also improve full-thickness wound healing in a mouse model. → PB-MSC secretome may promote cutaneous wound healing in horses.
Equine PB-MSC secretome	PB-MSC secretome inhibits biofilm formation and mature biofilms of *P aeruginosa, S aureus*, and *S epidermidis*. PB-MSC secretome also contains cysteine proteases that destabilize *MRSA* biofilms, making them more susceptible to antibiotic treatment. → PB-MSC secretome may inhibit biofilms in equine skin wounds.
Primary equine keratinocytes	Primary equine keratinocytes can be conditionally reprogrammed and then expanded in this undifferentiated state. They retain the ability to differentiate normally and form a stratified epithelium that may be appropriate for transplantation. → Keratinocytes can be expanded in culture to form material for skin grafts.
Equine PB-MSC secretome	PB-MSC secretome decreases the viability of *MRSA* biofilms in a skin biofilm explant model. CCL2 in CM increases the antimicrobial activity of equine keratinocytes by stimulating expression of AMPs. → PB-MSC secretome may inhibit *MRSA* growth and biofilms in equine skin wounds.

Abbreviations: AMPs, antimicrobial peptides; CCL2, CC motif chemokine ligand 2; DFs, dermal fibroblasts; *E coli*, *Escherichia coli*; EC, endothelial cells; EGT, exuberant granulation tissue; IGFBP-2, insulin-like growth factor binding protein 2; IL-8, interleukin 8; *MRSA*, methicillin-resistant *S aureus*; *P aeruginosa*, *Pseudomonas aeruginosa*; PAI-1, plasminogen activator inhibitor-1; PB-MSCs, peripheral blood-derived mesenchymal stromal cells; PDGF-AA, platelet-derived growth factor AA; *S aureus*, *Staphylococcus aureus*; *S epidermidis*, *Staphylococcus epidermidis*; VEGF-A, vascular endothelial growth factor A.

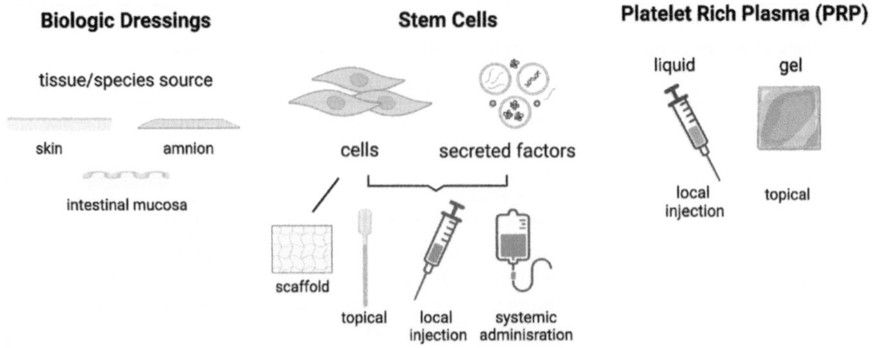

Fig. 5. Overview of biologic therapies and their potential delivery methods for treatment of equine cutaneous wounds.

This observation has prompted researchers to explore not only the efficacy of physical dressings to promote wound healing but also the effects of acellular products that can be extracted from dressing material on wounds.

Studies have been conducted to determine if equine amnion can serve as bandaging material for pinch-grafted wounds in ponies,[29] and if amnion or acellular amnion–derived products are effective at promoting distal wound healing in horses.[30–32] In the pony study, pinch-grafts, small disks of skin of ∼3 mm created by excising an elevated cone of skin,[33] were applied to experimentally induced full-thickness skin wounds on the limbs of 6 ponies. Half of the wounds were bandaged with amnion, the other half with a nonadherent wound dressing. Lost grafts and healing time were measured. The percentage of lost grafts did not differ between groups, but the median healing time for wounds bandaged with amnion (30 days) was significantly less compared to wounds bandaged with the nonadherent dressing (39 days). The authors concluded that amnion can be used for bandaging pinch-grafted wounds on the distal limbs of ponies.[29] Important to note is that his conclusion may not be applicable to horses, as distal limb wounds heal differently in ponies and horses.[13,34] In the earliest horse study, limb wounds were created on 9 animals and treated with either amnion or live yeast cell derivative beneath a nonadherent wound dressing. Nonadherent wound dressing alone was included as control. Rates of contraction and epithelialization were not different across groups. Throughout the study, however, the percentage of epithelialization was significantly greater and the severity of EGT was significantly less for wounds treated with amnion compared to the other 2 groups. Additionally, the number of days to complete healing was significantly less for wounds treated with amnion as compared to the other groups.[30] The objectives of a later horse study were to characterize the growth factors in a commercially available, injectable equine amniotic membrane product and to evaluate the effect of a related bandaging product on distal wound healing using an 8-horse cohort.[31] To meet the first objective, transforming growth factor (TGFβ1), vascular endothelial growth factor (VEGF), epidermal growth factor (EGF), platelet-derived growth factor (PDGF-BB), and prostaglandin E2 (PGE2) concentrations in the injectable product were assessed by enzyme-linked immunosorbent assay (ELSA). TGFβ1, VEGF, and PGE2 were detected; EGF and PDGF-BB concentrations were less than the lower limits of quantitation.[31] For the second objective, 2 full-thickness skin wounds were created on the forelimbs of each horse. Paired wounds on one limb were bandaged with the amnion-based product or left untreated. Paired wounds on the other limb were bandaged with a silicone dressing or left untreated. Read-outs were wound size and quality of wound healing based on histologic and immunohistochemistry assays. Treatment of wounds with the amnion-based product did not alter healing time based on wound size nor did it affect the quality of healing compared to other groups. Treatment was associated with increased granulation tissue production early in the study, which led the authors to determine that use of the product may be most beneficial for substantial wounds which require large amounts of granulation tissue to heal.[31] A more recent experiment was carried out to determine if a one-time injection of acellular amnion–derived components combined with amniotic fluid–derived products affected the healing time of experimentally created distal limb wounds, using 8 horses.[32] No difference in wound area was found between the treatment and control groups over time. The authors concluded that in the experimental model, a single treatment did not accelerate distal wound healing, but they proposed that naturally occurring chronic or nonhealing wounds may respond differently.[32]

In addition to amnion, other sources of biologic dressings have been tested. In a study consisting of 5 horses with experimentally created lower limb wounds, biologic dressings from 3 origins were applied: split-thickness allogeneic skin (composed of the epidermis and a portion of the dermis), allogeneic peritoneum, and xenogeneic porcine small intestinal submucosa.[35] When compared to wounds dressed with a nonadherent synthetic pad as control, no differences in bacterial proliferation, inflammation (based on histologic assessment), or vascularization were observed 6 days after application of the dressings. Healing time also did not differ across dressings. Based on these results, it was concluded that these biologic dressings do not offer advantages over a synthetic dressing for the treatment of small granulating wounds.[35]

Stem cells

Stem cells have been used for decades in equine medicine to treat joint and tendon injuries, with the first documented administration of MSCs into a lesion in the superficial digital flexor tendon of a horse in 2003.[36] Since then, larger and more complete orthopedic studies have been performed, and autologous MSCs are now routinely used clinically to treat orthopedic injuries.[37] In contrast, much less work has been done to determine if stem cells can also aid in the treatment of cutaneous wounds.

An early study involving 4 horses took advantage of naturally occurring limb wounds that were unresponsive to conventional therapies.[38] MSC-like cells derived from peripheral blood were injected at the wound sites, and wounds were visually assessed to evaluate wound healing parameters, including the formation of granulation tissue, crusts, and scars. The authors reported that all animals responded well to the cell injection, suggesting this might be a useful treatment for large wounds.[38] Members of the same group then went on to perform several additional small studies, using epithelial-like stem/progenitor cells (EpSCs) to treat experimentally induced skin wounds located dorsally from the *musculus gluteus medius*.[39–41] The first study involved 1 horse and was designed to compare the treatment of EpSCs combined with PRP to PRP alone.[39] Treatments were administered by an initial intradermal injection, followed by 2 topical treatments, with one immediately after injection and the other one 24 hours later. Histological parameters and wound sizes were assessed from biopsies collected 30 days post-treatment. Granulation tissue was restricted, and the dermis was thinner in the wounds treated with EpSCs plus PRP when compared to wounds treated with PRP alone. The EpSCs plus PRP-treated wounds also showed increased vascularization, elastin, and follicle-like structures, as well as a higher percentage of "filling" based on wound areas at day 30 when compared to wound areas immediately after wound creation. The authors concluded that EpSCs combined with PRP treatment led to microscopic and macroscopic improvements in wound healing parameters.[39] The second study was designed to compare autologous versus allogeneic EpSC treatment to (i) each other, (ii) a vehicle control, and (iii) an untreated control in a similar wound model, using 6 horses.[40] Wound exudates were evaluated on days 3, 7, and 14, and biopsies were taken at weeks 1, 2, and 5 to measure wound circumferences. The authors reported no differences across treatments in proinflammatory cytokines in exudates, nor in epidermal thickness, crust formation, dermoepidermal separation, epithelialization, edema, quantity and morphology of collagen, fibroblast maturation, granulation tissue morphology, and amount of immune cell infiltrates in the biopsies. The only reported difference was a significantly smaller circumference in autologous EpSC-treated wounds when compared to wounds treated with allogeneic EpSCs and control wounds. The authors concluded that both sources of EpSCs had similar effects but that more studies are warranted to confirm the clinical relevance of EpSCs as a wound treatment.[40] A follow-up experiment in 6 horses, using the same wound model and treatment groups, was carried out to look at mRNA expression at 1 and 5 weeks after treatment of growth factors and cytokines critical to successful wound healing, including epidermal keratin, EGF, VEGF, interferon gamma, and interleukin 6.[41] Although some differences in gene expression were found between the different treatment groups, no general conclusions were reported for this work.[41]

The potential of MSCs as a therapy for distal limb wounds has been explored by several groups in recent years.[42–44] The earliest study evaluated the effects of umbilical cord blood–derived MSCs (UCB-MSCs) in four forms: (i) normoxic- or (ii) hypoxic-preconditioned MSCs injected into wound margins, and (iii) normoxic- or (iv) hypoxic-preconditioned MSCs embedded in an autologous fibrin gel and applied topically to the wound bed. A saline-injected wound and a fibrin gel–treated wound served as controls. All treatments were administered to the distal limb wounds of 6 horses. Wound surface area, thermography, gene expression, and histologic scoring were evaluated weekly for 6 weeks. The results showed that both MSC treatments, irrespective of preconditioning, using the 2 different delivery methods were safe, improved histologic outcomes, and led to decreased wound area when compared to control wounds. Comparing the 2 delivery methods, wound areas were significantly decreased in wounds treated via injection when compared to topical application, and injection of MSCs also led to an increased gene expression of TGFβ1 and cyclooxygenase-2 expression 1 week after treatment. Also, significantly more wounds treated with MSCs were categorized as prohealing as opposed to proinflammatory histologically. Based on the outcomes, the authors concluded that UCB-MSCs are a promising therapy for distal extremity wounds when administered at wound margins via injection.[42]

A more recent experiment was designed to determine the extent of homing and engraftment of a high dose of intravenously (IV) administered fluorescently labeled allogeneic UCB-MSCs to surgically induced wounds on the forelimbs and thoraxes of 2 horses.[43] Wounds and contralateral nonwounded skin were biopsied on days 0, 1, 2, 7, 14, and 33 post-treatment. Findings confirmed that UCB-MSCs preferentially homed to wounds and persisted for at least 33 days post-treatment. The lack of adverse clinical effects led the group to conclude that the high dose of injected MSCs was safe. In addition, they stated that further studies are warranted to determine the effects of IV-administered UCB-MSCs on wound healing.[43]

Another recent study assessed the safety and clinical value of topically administered (i) allogeneic oral mucosa–derived MSCs (OM-MSCs) or (ii) the secretome of these OM-MSCs, each mixed in a hyaluronic acid (HA) gel, as treatments for experimentally induced distal forelimb and thorax wounds on 8 horses.[44] Controls consisted of no treatment and HA gel alone. Gross macroscopic evaluation was performed, and photographs were taken regularly to assess the surface area and additional features of the wounds. Biopsies representing normal skin were taken at each site before wound creation and compared to biopsies of wounds collected at day 62, after complete healing. Both OM-MSCs and the OM-MSC secretome had positive impacts on thorax wound contraction, and OM-MSCs improved contraction and epithelialization of forelimb wounds. Histological examination, however, revealed no significant differences between wound sites before and after treatment. The authors concluded that OM-MSCs and OM-MSC secretome combined with HA show a positive impact on healing when applied topically during the early stage of wounding.[44]

Platelet-rich plasma

PRP is an autologous treatment created by taking blood from a patient, removing cells other than platelets, followed by concentrating the platelets within the plasma fraction. As platelets secrete growth factors that trigger cell division and stimulate tissue regeneration, treating wounds with a concentrated platelet source may stimulate or speed up the healing process, decrease healing time, and minimize pain.[45–48] Similar to stem cells, PRP has been used to treat musculoskeletal injuries in horses for decades, and is only recently being explored as a therapy for cutaneous wound healing as well.[49]

Several published studies describe PRP as a therapy for surgically induced body wounds of horses.[50–52] In one study, surgical incisions were created on the necks of 6 horses that were either treated with a PRP gel or left untreated (control), and then sutured.[50] The major findings were that (i) untreated wounds displayed the most intense inflammatory responses; (ii) PRP-treated wounds had a keratinized stratified epithelium with normal morphology on day 5 postwounding that was not present in the controls; (iii) the dermis of the PRP-treated group exhibited organized interconnecting collagen fibers on day 15 postwounding, while the control had disorganized tissue at that time point; and (iv) the number of blood vessels was higher in the PRP-treated group as compared to the controls on days 30 and 45. Based on these findings, the authors concluded that PRP gel may serve as a practical and economical treatment for acute wounds.[50]

Another study focused specifically on surgically induced wounds in the gluteal region that were burned to create deep second-degree burns.[51] Four horses were divided into 2 treatment groups, with one group receiving one dose of autologous PRP gel applied topically under a bandage and the other group receiving the same treatment but then treated again 3 days later. Each treatment group included control wounds treated with saline solution in parallel. Biopsies were taken and examined by scanning electron microscopy on days 5, 15, 25, and 40 after the first treatment, and swabs were collected and plated for bacteria on day 30. Overall, an increased formation of fibrosis and a higher number of collagen fibrils were detected in PRP-treated wounds compared to the corresponding controls. Additional findings showed that 2 applications of PRP instead of one (i) accelerated ECM formation during early wound healing, (ii) led to fibril organization that was similar to uninjured tissue, and (iii) resulted in dense fibrotic tissue at day 40. Evidence of bacterial growth was observed in all groups, but no infection was detected. The authors concluded that PRP gel increases the rate of ECM repair, but with the potential to induce fibrosis, and provides antibacterial support, thus potentially preventing complications due to infection.[51]

An additional study evaluated the immunohistochemical expression of collagens during the healing process of skin treated with PRP.[52] Wounds created in the gluteal region of 7 horses were injected with PRP, and untreated wounds served as controls.

There was no significant difference in healing time between the treated and untreated groups. Biopsies were taken at day 14 postwounding and at wound closure. PRP-treated wounds showed better organization of bundled collagen fibers and contained more eosinophils when compared to controls. Collagen type 1 (COL1) staining was lower in the control group than in the treated group at day 14, but higher at wound closure; while Collagen type III (COLIII) was higher in the control group at day 14 and lower at wound closure. From this study, it was concluded that a single local treatment of PRP improves tissue quality, but that more in vivo studies are warranted to determine the effects of PRP on skin wound healing.[52]

PRP has also been tested as a treatment for distal limb wounds.[53–56] One clinical case study reports on the treatment of a chronic, severely contaminated distal limb wound of a foal via debridement, injection of autologous PRP, and bandaging.[53] No complications were observed as a result of the PRP treatment, and limb swelling diminished. Wound contraction and epithelization were noted at 8 days post-treatment, and the size of the wound had decreased by 50% after 2 weeks. Complete wound healing occurred 1 month post-treatment, and the foal fully recovered after 2 months. As no controls were included in this clinical case study, the authors hypothesized that PRP can be used as a treatment for severe distal limb wounds in horses but suggested that a controlled study should be performed to confirm this.[53] In another study, surgically induced wounds were created on the lower limbs of one horse and treated with PRP gel, saline, or left untreated.[54] Wounds were bandaged and treated again every 4 days for 24 days, and then every 8 days until day 79. Biopsies were taken at days 7, 36, and 79 postwounding. The overall results were that epithelial cells differentiated earlier in PRP-treated wounds when compared to control wounds, as supported by the accelerated expression of cytokeratin 10, and that PRP gel promoted the formation of organized collagen. These results prompted the authors to propose that PRP can induce wound repair in injuries previously deemed untreatable.[54] A larger study assessed the effects of PRP on 12 experimentally created distal forelimb wounds in 6 horses.[55] Half of the wounds were treated topically with 2 doses of PRP, while the other half received no treatment (controls). Macroscopic observations indicated that treated wounds took longer to heal than control wounds, but these differences were not significant after week 3. Histologically, no effects of the treatment were noted, and the strength of healed wound tissue did not differ based on treatment. TGFβ1 concentration was higher in treated wounds at week 1, but the difference was not significant, and no differences in *COL1* or *COLIII* mRNA expression were detected between treatment and control. The authors concluded that 2 topical applications of autologous PRP did not accelerate or improve healing of small, granulating, full-thickness wounds on limbs. However, as healing differs between small and large wounds,[57] and small wounds might potentially mask the detection of treatment effects, they suggested that PRP treatment may hold more promise for wounds with massive tissue loss or chronic wounds that could benefit from a fresh source of mediators to aid the healing process.[55]

A more recent experiment was designed to compare the effects of a single treatment of (i) autologous PRP injection, (ii) topical autologous PRP, (iii) allogeneic PRP injection, and (iv) saline injection as control, on the healing of surgically induced distal limb wounds.[56] Wounds were monitored daily for 15 days, and biopsies were collected at days 15 and 30 post-treatment. The overall findings were that (i) healing time was reduced in all treatment groups when compared to the control, (ii) moderate granulation tissue was observed in the control when compared to the treatment groups, (iii) autologous PRP injection led to mild inflammation and neovascularization,

(iv) allogeneic PRP injection did not cause local reactions, and (v) PRP gel had the most positive impacts on wound healing based on clinical and histopathological evaluations. These results led the authors to conclude that PRP in all forms had a positive impact on wound healing and thus warrants the need for future studies to further explore this treatment option.[56]

FUTURE DIRECTIONS

The overall conclusion from the case reports and small in vivo studies reviewed earlier, is that although biologic dressings and dressing products, stem cells, and PRP, show promise as treatment options for equine cutaneous wounds, larger, well-controlled trials are needed to confirm the efficacy of these therapies. Studies in horses are costly and labor intensive, so they should be well planned and based on evidence that the treatments to be tested will be effective. The latter can be gained from in vitro and/or ex vivo explant experiments, such as those outlined in **Table 1**. Additionally, studies focused on improving delivery methods and treatment schedules should direct the design of future in vivo trials designed to further optimize these biologic therapies promoting the healing of skin wounds of horses.

SUMMARY

Equine clinicians are increasingly interested in using biologics, including cell-based therapies, to treat cutaneous wounds of horses. In vitro studies have shown that MSCs secrete factors that promote wound healing and that primary keratinocytes can be reprogrammed to be used for transplantation. Small in vivo experiments suggest that biologic dressings and dressing products, stem cells, and PRP may promote skin wound healing. Delivery methods should be optimized, and larger trials are needed to confirm whether biologics do indeed improve skin wound healing in horses.

CLINICS CARE POINTS

- Healthy, uncompromised skin is required for the well-being of horses, making the treatment of skin wounds a high priority in equine medicine.
- Biologics, including stem cells and platelet rich plasma, have the potential to improve skin wound healing non-surgically, while reducing the need for conventional antibiotics.
- Methods for generating and delivering biologic therapies must be improved, and large clinical trials need to be conducted to confirm that these therapies are optimized to improve skin wound healing.

DISCLOSURE

The authors have no conflicts of interest to disclose.

ACKNOWLEDGMENTS

We would like to acknowledge the National Institute of Food and Agriculture, U.S. Department of Agriculture, who supports our equine MSC secretome studies through Competitive Grants no. 2018-67015-28309 and 2022-67015-36351. All figures were created with Biorender.com.

REFERENCES

1. Gould J. Superpowered skin. Nature 2018;563(7732):S84–5.
2. Cañedo-Dorantes L, Cañedo-Ayala M. Skin acute wound healing: a comprehensive review. Int J Inflamm 2019;2019:1–15.
3. Rodrigues M, Kosaric N, Bonham CA, et al. Wound healing: a cellular perspective. Physiol Rev 2019;99(1):665–706.
4. Theoret C, Schumacher J, editors. Equine wound management. Third edition. Ames, IA, USA: Wiley Blackwell; 2017. p. 369–84.
5. Theoret CL, Wilmink JM. Aberrant wound healing in the horse: Naturally occurring conditions reminiscent of those observed in man: Wound healing in the horse reminiscent of healing in man. Wound Repair Regen 2013;21(3):365–71.
6. Higgins G, Martin S. Horse anatomy for performance. Pynes Hill, Exeter, UK: David & Charles; 2012.
7. Gerber PA, Buhren BA, Schrumpf H, et al. The top skin-associated genes: a comparative analysis of human and mouse skin transcriptomes. Biol Chem 2014;395(6):577–91.
8. Theoret CL, Olutoye OO, Parnell LKS, et al. Equine exuberant granulation tissue and human keloids: a comparative histopathologic study: Equine Exuberant Granulation Tissue and Human Keloids. Vet Surg 2013. https://doi.org/10.1111/j.1532-950X.2013.12055.x.
9. Lepault E, Céleste C, Doré M, et al. Comparative study on microvascular occlusion and apoptosis in body and limb wounds in the horse. Wound Repair Regen 2005;13(5):520–9.
10. Celeste CJ, Deschene K, Riley CB, et al. Regional differences in wound oxygenation during normal healing in an equine model of cutaneous fibroproliferative disorder: Regional differences in oxygenation in equine wounds. Wound Repair Regen 2011;19(1):89–97.
11. Celeste CJ, Deschesne K, Riley CB, et al. Skin temperature during cutaneous wound healing in an equine model of cutaneous fibroproliferative disorder: kinetics and anatomic-site differences. Vet Surg 2013;42(2):147–53.
12. Eggleston RB. Wound Management. Vet Clin North Am Equine Pract 2018;34(3):511–38.
13. Wilmink JM, van Weeren PR. Second-intention repair in the horse and pony and management of exuberant granulation tissue. Vet Clin North Am Equine Pract 2005;21(1):15–32.
14. Jacobs KA, Leach DH, Fretz PB, et al. Comparative aspects of the healing of excisional wounds on the leg and body of horses. Vet Surg 2008;13(2):83–90.
15. Jørgensen E, Bjarnsholt T, Jacobsen S. Biofilm and equine limb wounds. Animals 2021;11(10):2825.
16. Raidal S. Antimicrobial stewardship in equine practice. Aust Vet J 2019;97(7):238–42.
17. Russell KA, Garbin LC, Wong JM, et al. Mesenchymal stromal cells as potential antimicrobial for veterinary use—a comprehensive review. Front Microbiol 2020;11:606404.
18. World Health Organization. *Antimicrobial resistance: global report on surveillance*. Geneva: World Health Organization; 2014. https://apps.who.int/iris/handle/10665/112642.
19. Battah B. Mesenchymal stem cells: potential role against bacterial infection. J Basic Microbiol 2022;10(03):97–113.

20. Bussche L, Van de Walle GR. Peripheral blood-derived mesenchymal stromal cells promote angiogenesis via paracrine stimulation of vascular endothelial growth factor secretion in the equine model. Stem Cells Transl Med 2014;3(12):1514–25.
21. Bussche L, Harman RM, Syracuse BA, et al. Microencapsulated equine mesenchymal stromal cells promote cutaneous wound healing in vitro. Stem Cell Res Ther 2015;6:66.
22. Harman RM, Bihun IV, Van de Walle GR. Secreted factors from equine mesenchymal stromal cells diminish the effects of TGF-β1 on equine dermal fibroblasts and alter the phenotype of dermal fibroblasts isolated from cutaneous fibroproliferative wounds: Mesenchymal stromal cell effects on fibroblasts. Wound Repair Regen 2017. https://doi.org/10.1111/wrr.12515.
23. Harman RM, Yang S, He MK, et al. Antimicrobial peptides secreted by equine mesenchymal stromal cells inhibit the growth of bacteria commonly found in skin wounds. Stem Cell Res Ther 2017;8(1). https://doi.org/10.1186/s13287-017-0610-6.
24. Harman RM, He MK, Zhang S, et al. Plasminogen activator inhibitor-1 and tenascin-C secreted by equine mesenchymal stromal cells stimulate dermal fibroblast migration in vitro and contribute to wound healing in vivo. Cytotherapy 2018. https://doi.org/10.1016/j.jcyt.2018.06.005.
25. Marx C, Gardner S, Harman RM, et al. The mesenchymal stromal cell secretome impairs methicillin-resistant *Staphylococcus aureus* biofilms via cysteine protease activity in the equine model: Biofilm impairment via MSC-secreted proteases. STEM CELLS Transl Med 2020. https://doi.org/10.1002/sctm.19-0333.
26. Alkhilaiwi F, Wang L, Zhou D, et al. Long-term expansion of primary equine keratinocytes that maintain the ability to differentiate into stratified epidermis. Stem Cell Res Ther 2018;9(1). https://doi.org/10.1186/s13287-018-0918-x.
27. Marx C, Gardner S, Harman RM, et al. Mesenchymal stromal cell-secreted CCL2 promotes antibacterial defense mechanisms through increased antimicrobial peptide expression in keratinocytes. Stem Cells Transl Med 2021;10(12):1666–79.
28. Pruitt BA. Characteristics and uses of biologic dressings and skin substitutes. Arch Surg 1984;119(3):312.
29. Goodrich LR, Moll HD, Crisman MV, et al. Comparison of equine amnion and a nonadherent wound dressing material for bandaging pinch-grafted wounds in ponies. AJVR (Am J Vet Res) 2000;61(3):326–9.
30. Bigbie RB, Schumacher J, Swaim SF, et al. Effects of amnion and live yeast cell derivative on second-intention healing in horses. Am J Vet Res 1991;52(8):1376–82.
31. Fowler AW, Gilbertie JM, Watson VE, et al. Effects of acellular equine amniotic allografts on the healing of experimentally induced full-thickness distal limb wounds in horses. Vet Surg 2019;48(8):1416–28.
32. Duddy HR, Schoonover MJ, Williams MR, et al. Healing time of experimentally induced distal limb wounds in horses is not reduced by local injection of equine-origin liquid amnion allograft. AJVR (Am J Vet Res) 2022;83(8). https://doi.org/10.2460/ajvr.21.10.0169. ajvr.21.10.0169.
33. Schumacher J, Hanselka DV. Skin Grafting of the Horse. Vet Clin North Am Equine Pract 1989;5(3):591–614.
34. Wilmink JM, Stolk PW, van Weeren PR, et al. Differences in second-intention wound healing between horses and ponies: macroscopic aspects. Equine Vet J 1999;31(1):53–60.

35. Gomez JH, Schumacher J, Lauten SD, et al. Effects of 3 biologic dressings on healing of cutaneous wounds on the limbs of horses. Can J Vet Res 2004; 68(1):49–55.
36. Smith RKW, Korda M, Blunn GW, et al. Isolation and implantation of autologous equine mesenchymal stem cells from bone marrow into the superficial digital flexor tendon as a potential novel treatment. Equine Vet J 2003;35(1):99–102.
37. Gerth AG, Oldak T, Baran J, et al. Mesenchymal stem cells for orthopedic treatments and regenerative medicine. Stem Cells Translational Medicine 2019; 8(S1):S15.
38. Spaas JH, Broeckx S, Walle GR, et al. The effects of equine peripheral blood stem cells on cutaneous wound healing: a clinical evaluation in four horses. Clin Exp Dermatol 2013;38(3):280–4.
39. Broeckx SY, Maes S, Martinello T, et al. Equine epidermis: a source of epithelial-like stem/progenitor cells with in vitro and in vivo regenerative capacities. Stem Cell Dev 2014;23(10):1134–48.
40. Broeckx SY, Borena BM, Van Hecke L, et al. Comparison of autologous versus allogeneic epithelial-like stem cell treatment in an in vivo equine skin wound model. Cytotherapy 2015;17(10):1434–46.
41. Spaas JH, Gomiero C, Broeckx SY, et al. Wound-healing markers after autologous and allogeneic epithelial-like stem cell treatment. Cytotherapy 2016;18(4): 562–9.
42. Textor JA, Clark KC, Walker NJ, et al. Allogeneic stem cells alter gene expression and improve healing of distal limb wounds in horses: stem cell treatment of wounds in horses. STEM CELLS Translational Medicine 2018;7(1):98–108.
43. Mund SJK, Kawamura E, Awang-Junaidi AH, et al. Homing and engraftment of intravenously administered equine cord blood-derived multipotent mesenchymal stromal cells to surgically created cutaneous wound in horses: a pilot project. Cells 2020;9(5):1162.
44. Di Francesco P, Cajon P, Desterke C, et al. Effect of allogeneic oral mucosa mesenchymal stromal cells on equine wound repair. Vet Med Int 2021;2021: 1–10. https://doi.org/10.1155/2021/5024905. Hikasa Y.
45. Chicharro-Alcántara D, Rubio-Zaragoza M, Damiá-Giménez E, et al. Platelet rich plasma: new insights for cutaneous wound healing management. J Forensic Biomech 2018;9(1):10.
46. Barrionuevo DV, Laposy CB, Abegão KGB, et al. Comparison of experimentally-induced wounds in rabbits treated with different sources of platelet-rich plasma. Lab Anim 2015;49(3):209–14.
47. Lai CY, Li TY, Lam KHS, et al. The long-term analgesic effectiveness of platelet-rich plasma injection for carpal tunnel syndrome: a cross-sectional cohort study. Pain Med 2022;23(7):1249–58.
48. Cook JL, Smith PA, Bozynski CC, et al. Multiple injections of leukoreduced platelet rich plasma reduce pain and functional impairment in a canine model of ACL and meniscal deficiency: PRP IN ACL, MENISCAL HEALING. J Orthop Res 2016;34(4):607–15.
49. Brossi PM, Moreira JJ, Machado TS, et al. Platelet-rich plasma in orthopedic therapy: a comparative systematic review of clinical and experimental data in equine and human musculoskeletal lesions. BMC Vet Res 2015;11(1):98.
50. DeRossi R, Coelho ACA de O, Mello GS de, et al. Effects of platelet-rich plasma gel on skin healing in surgical wound in horses. Acta Cir Bras 2009;24(4):276–81.

51. Maciel FB, DeRossi R, Módolo TJC, et al. Scanning electron microscopy and microbiological evaluation of equine burn wound repair after platelet-rich plasma gel treatment. Burns 2012;38(7):1058–65.
52. Souza MV de, Silva MB, Pinto J de O, et al. Immunohistochemical expression of collagens in the skin of horses treated with leukocyte-poor platelet-rich plasma. BioMed Res Int 2015;2015:1–12.
53. López C, Carmona JU. Platelet-rich plasma as an adjunctive therapy for the management of a severe chronic distal limb wound in a foal. J Equine Vet Sci 2014; 34(9):1128–33.
54. Carter CA, Jolly DG, Worden CE, et al. Platelet-rich plasma gel promotes differentiation and regeneration during equine wound healing. Exp Mol Pathol 2003; 74(3):244–55.
55. Monteiro SO, Lepage OM, Theoret CL. Effects of platelet-rich plasma on the repair of wounds on the distal aspect of the forelimb in horses. Am J Vet Res 2009;70(2):277–82.
56. Pereira RC da F, De La Côrte FD, Brass KE, et al. Evaluation of three methods of platelet-rich plasma for treatment of equine distal limb skin wounds. J Equine Vet Sci 2019;72:1–7.
57. Berry DB II, Sullins KE. Effects of topical application of antimicrobials and bandaging on healing and granulation tissue formation in wounds of the distal aspect of the limbs in horses. AJVR (Am J Vet Res) 2003;64(1):88–92.

Use of Biologics and Stem Cells in Equine Ophthalmology

Brian Christopher Gilger, DVM, MS, Dipl ACVO, Dipl ABT

KEYWORDS

- Equine • Eye • Stem cells • Gene therapy • Biologics

KEY POINTS

- Topically applied biologics, such as platelet-rich plasma, may improve the healing of corneal ulcers and reduce inflammation.
- Amniotic membrane grafts may improve corneal wound healing by providing anti-inflammatory, antifibrosis, and protective (ie, bandage) effects.
- Local or systemic mesenchymal stem cells have wound healing and immunomodulating effects that may be used therapeutically for the treatment of keratitis, uveitis, and ocular posterior segment diseases.
- Immunomodulatory transgenes and other biologics transferred by viral vectors (gene therapy) may be effective in the treatment of equine uveitis.

INTRODUCTION

The purpose of this article is to describe the potential of regenerative therapies for the equine eye. Because of the high rate of ocular injury, infections, and immunologic conditions in the horse, there is a significant unmet need for efficacious, practical, and safe therapies for equine ocular diseases. Of particular concern are the equine keratoapathies, such as non-healing corneal ulceration (eg, indolent corneal ulcers), infectious keratitis (eg, fungal and bacterial), and immune-mediated keratitis. Treatment for these conditions consists currently of the use of frequent, long-term, topical ocular, and systemic therapies. These can be difficult to administer, resulting in poor treatment compliance, toxic side effects, and poor efficacy, leading in many cases to blindness and loss of the globe. Another area of concern where there are few effective treatment options is equine uveitis. Like equine keratopathies, uveitis requires long-term and frequent medical therapy with high rates of treatment failure and subsequent blindness.

There are several clinical reports of the use of biologics and regenerative therapies for equine ophthalmic diseases. Unfortunately, most of these reports are case series

North Carolina State University, 1060 William Moore Drive, Raleigh, NC 27607, USA
E-mail address: bgilger@ncsu.edu

Vet Clin Equine 39 (2023) 541–552
https://doi.org/10.1016/j.cveq.2023.06.004
vetequine.theclinics.com

and not carefully controlled studies.[1–7] The studies, however, demonstrate promise for the use of regenerative and biological therapy for equine ocular diseases. In particular, the use of topical blood products such as serum, plasma, and platelet-rich plasma (PRP) or amniotic membrane (or derivatives) may have a positive therapeutic effect on the healing of stubborn corneal ulcers. Also, the use of mesenchymal stem cells and their immunomodulating properties may be effective in the treatment of corneal ulcers and immune-mediated keratitis (IMMK). Similarly, local therapy of mesenchymal stem cells or immunosuppressive gene therapy for equine recurrent uveitis may provide long-term effective treatments for this challenging disease.

In the article, we will review the regenerative and biologic therapies described for use in various anatomical areas of the equine eye including ocular surface, corneal, uveal, and ocular posterior segment diseases.

CORNEAL ULCERATION

Infectious keratitis and superficial non-healing corneal ulcers are the most common ocular diseases in horses.[8] Use of various autologous and non-autologous blood products, such as serum and plasma have been applied topically to horses for years (**Table 1**).[8–10] Use of topical serum to provide anti-collagenase activity to prevent corneal damage during bacterial infectious has been widely studied.[11,12] Use of anti-collagenase helps to prevent corneal enzymatic destruction or melting, which is particularly common in *pseudomonas spp* corneal infections (**Fig. 1**). The frequency of topical autologous serum is similar to that of topical antibiotics, with increased application frequency with more severe or advanced diseases. One study demonstrated that serum was equally efficacious as tetanus antitoxin and acetylcysteine to protect corneas from collagenase digestion.[12] Conway and colleagues,[11] demonstrated that fresh plasma has similar anti-collagenase efficacy in horse cornea compared to serum *in vitro*, and suggested that plasma would be an acceptable substitute for serum in the topical treatment of keratomalacia.[11] Although topical serum and plasma may be efficacious in horses with infection-related enzymatic damage to the corneal stroma, there have been no studies to date that demonstrate enhanced healing or re-epithelization of equine corneal ulcers with the use of topical serum. Furthermore, no improved epithelial healing rates were observed with the use of topical serum in a recent study of superficial non-healing corneal ulcers in dogs.[13]

Plasma-rich plasma (PRP), plasma rich in growth factors (PRGF), and serum from platelet-rich fibrin (s-PRF-drops) have increased concentrations of pro-epithelialization factors such as transforming growth factor (TGF)-β1, epidermal growth factor (EGF), and fibronectin compared to serum.[14] These substances have been evaluated *in vitro* or *in vivo* for their effect on equine corneal cells or corneal wound healing in horses, respectively (see **Table 1**).[15,16] In an *in vitro* study which compared PRP to PRGF and serum-treated cells, corneal stromal and limbal cells had enhanced proliferation and migration when treated with PRP, PRGF-treated cells had persistent cell proliferation but no improved migration, while serum-treated cells had a reduction in proliferation but an improvement in migration (see **Table 1**).[15] In humans, both fresh or stored (4 weeks at 4C) PRP eye drops were shown to significantly improve corneal epithelial wound healing *in vivo* compared with PBS or autologous serum.[14] Although equine clinical studies on the use of PRP for the treatment of corneal ulceration have not been reported, these studies provide support for the clinical evaluation of topical ocular use of PRP in horses for improved healing of corneal ulceration. However, a study in donkeys demonstrated no significant effect on experimental corneal wound healing with topically applied s-PRF-drops.[16]

Table 1
Biologic use for corneal ulceration in horses

Corneal Disease	Biologic Used	*In vitro* or *in vivo*	Effect	Reference
Keratomalacia (melting)	Serum	*In vitro*	Prevent collagenase corneal destruction; improved epithelial cell migration	Haffner et al,[12] 2003 & Conway, et al,[11] 2016 Rushton, et al,[15] 2018
	Plasma	*In vitro*	Prevent collagenase corneal destruction	Conway, et al,[11] 2016
	Amnion membrane graft	*In vivo*	Successful healing of keratomalacia	Lassaline, et al,[1] 2005 Plummer, et al,[2] 2009
Ulcerative keratitis	Plasma-rich plasma (PRP)	*In vitro*	Improved corneal epithelial cell proliferation and migration	Rushton, et al,[15] 2018
	Plasma rich in growth factors (PRGF)	*In vitro*	Constant corneal epithelial cell proliferation, no improvement in migration	Rushton, et al,[15] 2018
	Serum from platelet-rich fibrin (s-PRF-drops)	*In vivo* (experimental in donkeys)	No significant effect on corneal wound healing	Hosny, et al,[16] 2022
	Equine umbilical cord serum (UCS),	*In vivo* (clinical)	Successful healing of diverse array of keratitis	Peyrecave-Capo, et al,[5] 2022
	Amniotic membrane suspension	*Ex vivo* culture model (rabbit)	Area and opacity of corneal wound decreased, but not ulcer	Boss, et al,[19] 2022
	Amniotic membrane extract	*In vivo,* experimental horses	No differences detected in the rate of epithelialization compared to controls	Lyons, et al,[18] 2021
	Autologous bone-marrow-derived mesenchymal stem cells (BM-MSCs)	*In vitro,* equine corneal stromal cells	Improved experimental healing	Sherman, et al,[20] 2017
	Blood-derived stem cells (BDSC)	*In vivo,* clinical cases	Clinical improvement in 2 cases with chronic ulcerative keratitis	Marfe, et al,[4] 2012

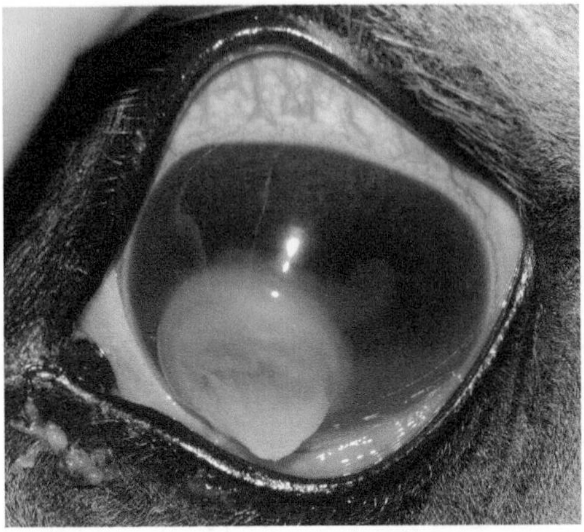

Fig. 1. Enzymatic, collagenase destruction or melting of the cornea in a horse with *pseudomonas spp* corneal infection.

Equine umbilical cord serum (UCS), which reportedly has high concentrations of insulin growth factor, transforming growth factor-beta 1 (TGF-β1), and platelet-derived growth factor but is largely devoid of pro-inflammatory cytokines, was used topically in six diverse infectious and non-infectious ulcerative keratopathies (see **Table 1**).[5] Along with standard ulcer treatment, UCS was applied topically 3 times a day for up to 15 days without observed adverse effects. All corneas eventually healed, but without controls, the beneficial effect of the UCS on healing is difficult to determine.[5]

Amnion membrane grafts or amniotic membrane extracts have been used for the treatment of horses with pseudomonas-associated keratomalacia and bullous keratopathy (**Fig. 2**, see **Table 1**),[1,2] and as an adjunct procedure with penetrating keratoplasty or keratectomy (for the treatment of neoplasia or IMMK).[2,3] Amniotic membranes are thought to enhance wound healing through inherent anti-angiogenic, anti-inflammatory, and antifibrosis factors[2,17] and by providing mechanical support and hydration to the cornea (ie, bandage effect). Amnion is thought to modulate TGF-β signaling and provide hepatocyte, epidermal, and keratocyte growth factors,

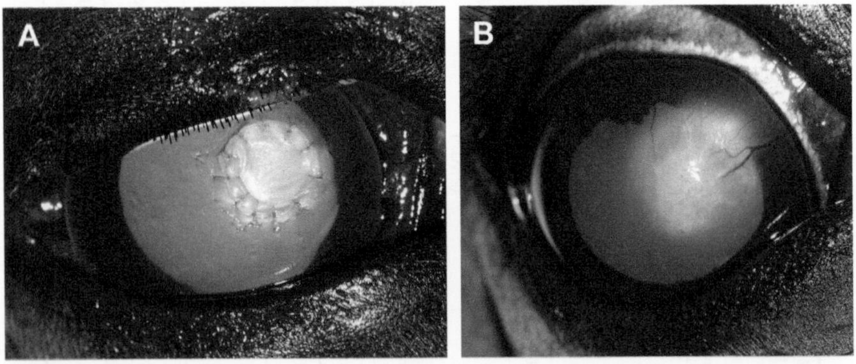

Fig. 2. Amnion membrane grafts. (*A*). Immediate post-operative placement of an amniotic membrane graft for the treatment of a melting ulcer. (*B*). Four weeks after surgery, the graft has vascularized and the keratitis is resolving.

which work together to reduce both scar formation and the expression of inflammatory cytokines.[2,17] Use of amniotic membranes, however, requires surgical intervention generally consisting of a keratectomy or extensive debridement, depending on the corneal disease, and requires sutures or a biologic adhesive to secure it to the ocular surface.

To avoid general anesthesia and corneal scarring associated with suture placement in amniotic membrane grafts, amniotic membrane extract or suspensions have been developed to be administered topically to horses for the treatment of ulcerative keratitis (see **Table 1**).[18,19] However, corneal epithelization rates in an air-liquid interface *ex vivo* rabbit corneal culture model did not differ between corneas treated with topical equine amniotic membrane suspension vs media controls, but area and intensity of corneal wound opacity were significantly reduced in corneas treated with the equine amniotic membrane suspension.[19] Similarly, in experimental horses, 8 mm corneal epithelial ulcers were treated topically with either a commercial amniotic membrane extract or a vehicle. There were no differences detected in the rate of epithelialization between the amniotic membrane extract-treated eyes and controls.[18] Use of amniotic membrane extract has not been reported in clinical cases, where there may be a beneficial therapeutic effect when there is the presence of keratomalacia or infection.

Autologous bone-marrow-derived mesenchymal stem cells (BM-MSCs) were shown to improve experimental healing of corneal stromal cells in an *in vitro* scratch assay compared to mesenchymal stem cell supernatant (MSC-Sp) or media controls (see **Table 1**).[20] Furthermore, MSC-Sp improved the closure of the scratch assay wound compared to media alone.[20] The conclusion of this study was that both the BM-MSCs and MSC-Sp may be effective in improving the healing of corneal ulceration in horses. Although the use of BM-MSC for the treatment of corneal ulceration has not been reported, the use of blood-derived stem cells (BDSC) administered intravenously and locally (either by eyedrops or subconjunctival injection) appeared to be associated with clinical improvement in two horses with chronic corneal ulceration (see **Table 1**).[4]

IMMUNE-MEDIATED KERATITIS

Immune-mediated keratitis (IMMK) is a chronic and relapsing corneal inflammatory disease associated with a variable degree of corneal cellular infiltration and vascularization, however, it is generally associated with little ocular discomfort unless there is corneal ulceration, bullous keratopathy, or corneal degeneration accompanying the disease.[21] The underlying causes of IMMK are likely heterogeneous, however, the pathogenesis is immunologic.[22] Current treatment of IMMK consists of frequent topical application of corticosteroids and immunosuppressant medications such as cyclosporine.[23] Although effective at controlling the disease in most cases, the treatment is lifelong and prone to poor compliance and disease recurrence. In some cases, the disease progresses to complete corneal opacity and blindness. Therefore, there is a significant unmet need for improved and practical therapies for IMMK.

In addition to their tissue regenerative properties, equine mesenchymal stem cells (MSCs) are known to modulate the immune response by reducing lymphocyte proliferation and inflammatory cytokine production. Additionally, MSCs have been shown in animal models to decrease corneal surface inflammation, neovascularization, and opacification,[24–27] all common clinical manifestations of equine IMMK.[21,22] Subconjunctival injection of autologous BM-MSCs was evaluated in a series of horses with IMMK (**Table 2**).[7] One ml of BM-MSCs (15 million cells/mL) suspended in autologous serum was injected under the bulbar conjunctiva either once or repeated approximately every 3-4 weeks for 3-5 injections in 4 cases of IMMK (**Fig. 3**). Three of 4 horses had

Table 2
Biologic use for immune-mediated keratitis in horses

Corneal Disease	Biologic Used	*In vitro* or *in vivo*	Effect	Reference
Immune-mediated keratitis	Autologous BM-MSCs	*In vivo* (15 million cells/injection) subconjunctivally (single or repeated doses)	Clinical resolution in 3 of 4 cases without recurrence	Davis, et al,[7] 2019
Immune mediated keratitis	Autologous BDSC	In vivo, Intravenously and locally (subconjunctivally)	Single case, improvement within 2 weeks	Marfe, et al,[4] 2012

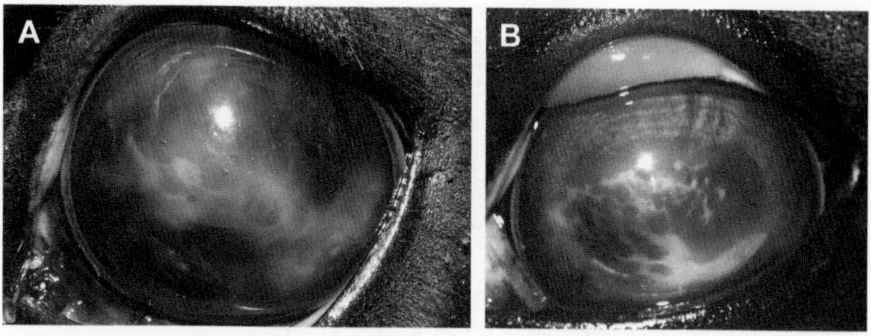

Fig. 3. Immune mediate keratitis (IMMK) treated with subconjunctival bone-marrow-derived mesenchymal stem cells (BM-MSCs). (*A*). Chronic IMMK with characteristic signs of corneal vascularization, corneal opacity, fibrosis, and early calcific keratopathy. (*B*). the Same eye 6 weeks later immediately following of the final dose of a series of 3 subconjunctival injections of 15 million BM-MSCs cells. Note the keratitis has nearly resolved with corneal fibrosis and scarring evident.

complete resolution without recurrence of the disease, while one horse had no observable clinical effect of the BM-MSCs.[7] In another study, autologous BDSC was injected intravenously and locally (subconjunctivally) in a case of IMMK and within 2 weeks, there were signs of improvement without reported relapse (see **Table 2**).[4] Number of BDSC used at each site of injection and if there were any associated adverse effects were not reported.[4]

UVEITIS AND OCULAR POSTERIOR SEGMENT DISEASE

Although uveitis can be secondary to infectious disease and keratopathies, the chronic and relapsing nature of recurrent uveitis (ERU) is the most difficult to treat (**Fig. 4**). Equine recurrent uveitis is a spontaneous, painful, and vision-threatening non-infectious in horses. It is characterized by episodes of active ocular inflammation alternating with varying intervals of clinical quiescence.[28–30] The accumulated effects

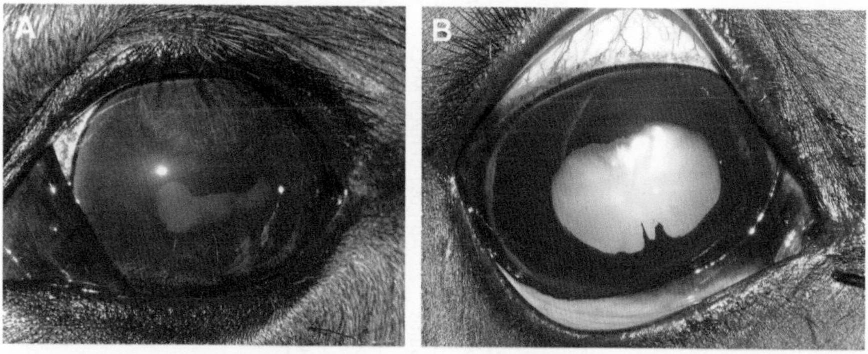

Fig. 4. Equine recurrent uveitis. (*A*). Active bout of inflammation in uveitis. Active uveitis is evident with corneal haze, anterior chamber fibrin formation, miosis, and swelling of the iris. (*B*). Chronic uveitis following multiple bouts of inflammation. Common clinical signs of chronic uveitis in horses include hyperpigmented iris, posterior synechia, corpora nigra atrophy, and cataract formation.

Table 3
Biologic use for uveitis and ocular posterior segment disease in the horse

Ocular Disease	Biologic Used	*In vitro* or *in vivo*	Effect	Reference
Recurrent uveitis	Adipose-derived MSCs	*In vitro*	Co-culture of MSCs with ERU CD + T cells decreased markers of activation	Saldinger, et al,[6] 2020
Recurrent uveitis	Adipose-derived MSCs	*In vivo*, Intravenous	Injections are safe, but therapeutic response not reported	Saldinger, et al,[6] 2020 Kol, et al,[31] 2015
Recurrent uveitis	Adeno-associated virus equine IL10	*In vivo*, experimental uveitis model	Intravitreal injection of AAV-eqIL10 eliminated the development of experimental immunologic uveitis	Crabtree, et al,[37] 2022
Retinal detachment	Autologous BDSC	*In vivo*, Intravenously	Vision was regained 3 months after treatment	Marfe, et al,[4] 2012

of recurrent "bouts" or "flares" of inflammation lead to progressively destructive pathologic changes including irreversible scarring, ocular cloudiness, cataract formation, and vision loss. Conventional treatment of ERU is non-specific, including frequent use of topical and systemic corticosteroids and other topical or oral immunosuppressive agents; none of which are effective in preventing uveitis relapses.[28,30] These therapies are limited by poor treatment compliance and long-term adverse effects, such as corneal degeneration, glaucoma, cataract, ocular hypertension, and infection, all of which may contribute to the development of blindness.[28]

As mentioned above, the known immunomodulating properties of stem cells may lend them to be effective in the treatment of equine uveitis and ERU (**Table 3**).[28,29] In a recent study, CD4+ T-cells from ERU horses expressed higher levels of interferon-gamma (IFNγ) than cells from control horses indicative of a shift toward a Th1 activation phenotype.[6] Co-incubation of these ERU-derived CD4+ T-cells with fat-derived MSCs significantly decreased markers of T-cell activation including decreased intracellular IFNγ, intracellular FoxP3, and surface CD25.[6] These data support the further evaluation of MSCs for the management of ERU. Furthermore, intravenous use of adipose-derived stem cells for the treatment of clinical cases of ERU has been described.[6] Although the clinical effect of the MSCs on ERU was not reported, the use of repeated intravenous MSCs in horses was well tolerated and did not induce system inflammation (see **Table 3**).[6,31]

Gene therapy is being developed for specific targeted therapy of a variety of ocular diseases including inherited retinal diseases.[32–34] Viral vectors are used to introduce DNA of missing molecules (due to a genetic defect) or therapeutic transgenes to affected tissues. One interesting transgene that may be effective in equine ocular disease is the immunomodulatory cytokine, interleukin-10 (IL-10). IL-10 has potent anti-inflammatory and immunomodulating properties that play critical roles in limiting the immune response and preventing autoimmune disorders.[35,36] IL-10 plays an important role in uveitis by protecting the eye from chronic inflammation and help preventing relapses of inflammation, thus suggesting that the ocular supplementation of endogenous IL-10 may be a promising therapeutic for ERU. A recent study demonstrated that equine IL-10 DNA delivered using the adeno-associated virus (AAV) gene therapy vector was safe and effective in inhibiting uveitis in an experimental autoimmune uveitis rat model (see **Table 3**).[37] Further studies are needed in the horse to determine the effective dose to transduce relevant equine ocular tissues and to determine safety. However, if effective, this gene therapy could eliminate ERU with a single ocular injection.

RETINAL DETACHMENT

Intravenous MSCs reportedly can migrate to sites of inflammation and exert a local anti-inflammatory and immunomodulating effect.[6,31,38] Therefore, the use of IV MSCs to treat ocular posterior segment diseases (ie, disease of the choroid, retina, and optic nerve) seems plausible. One report describes the use of autologous BDSC was injected intravenously in a horse with a bilateral retinal detachment of unknown cause. Three months after the IV administration of BDSCs, the horse reportedly regained vision in one eye (see **Table 3**).[4] Despite these promising results, further study is needed to optimize the route of therapy, dose, and type of MSC for the treatment of ocular posterior segment disease in horses.

SUMMARY

The use of regenerative medicine and biologics in equine ophthalmology is in its infancy, however, studies reported to date, both *in vitro* and *in vivo*, show promising results that warrant further investigation for use in the treatment of equine ocular disease. Of particular interest and promise is the use of PRP in ocular surface disease to improve corneal wound healing, the use of MSCs for immunomodulating properties for the treatment of ocular surface diseases such as IMMK, and the use of gene therapy to deliver biologics for diseases such as ERU. Much work remains to be done to determine optimal routes of therapy, the long-term efficacy, and the side effects of the use of these therapies in the equine eye.

CLINICS CARE POINTS

- Use of PRP in ocular surface disease to improve corneal wound healing and the use of MSCs for immunomodulating properties for the treatment of ocular surface diseases such as IMMK, appear very feasible in practice.
- Use of gene therapy to deliver biologics for diseases such as ERU is being developed.
- Much work remains to be done to determine optimal routes of therapy, the long-term efficacy, and the side effects of the use of these therapies in the equine eye.

DISCLOSURE

The author is listed on a provisional patent (PCT/US2022/027283), owned by NC State University, for the use of gene therapy for ocular diseases in horses. The author is a co-founder of Astro Therapeutics and Bedrock Therapeutics which are developing immunosuppressive gene therapy for ocular use.

REFERENCES

1. Lassaline ME, Brooks DE, Ollivier FJ, et al. Equine amniotic membrane transplantation for corneal ulceration and keratomalacia in three horses. Vet Ophthalmol 2005;8(5):311–7.
2. Plummer CE. The use of amniotic membrane transplantation for ocular surface reconstruction: a review and series of 58 equine clinical cases (2002–2008). Vet Ophthalmol 2009;12:17–24.
3. Ollivier F, Kallberg M, Plummer C, et al. Amniotic membrane transplantation for corneal surface reconstruction after excision of corneolimbal squamous cell carcinomas in nine horses. Vet Ophthalmol 2006;9(6):404–13.
4. Marfe G, Massaro-Giordano M, Ranalli M, et al. Blood derived stem cells: an ameliorative therapy in veterinary ophthalmology. J Cell Physiol 2012;227(3):1250–6.
5. Peyrecave-Capo X, Saulnier N, Maddens S, et al. Equine umbilical cord serum composition and its healing effects in equine corneal ulceration, *Front Vet Sci*, 9, 2022, 1-12.
6. Saldinger LK, Nelson SG, Bellone RR, et al. Horses with equine recurrent uveitis have an activated CD4+ T-cell phenotype that can be modulated by mesenchymal stem cells in vitro. Vet Ophthalmol 2020;23(1):160–70.
7. Davis AB, Schnabel LV, Gilger BC. Subconjunctival bone marrow-derived mesenchymal stem cell therapy as a novel treatment alternative for equine immune-mediated keratitis: a case series. Vet Ophthalmol 2019;22(5):674–82.
8. Brooks DE, Plummer CE. *Diseases of the Equine Cornea*. In: Gilger BC, editor. *Equine Ophthalmology*. 4th edition; 2022. p. 253–440.

9. Ollivier F, Gilger B, Barrie K, et al. Proteinases of the cornea and preocular tear film. Vet Ophthalmol 2007;10(4):199–206.
10. Clode A. Therapy of equine infectious keratitis: a review. Equine Vet J 2010; 42(S37):19–23.
11. Conway ED, Stiles J, Townsend WM, et al. Comparison of the in vitro anticollagenase efficacy of homologous serum and plasma on degradation of corneas of cats, dogs, and horses. Am J Vet Res 2016;77(6):627–33.
12. Haffner JC, Fecteau KA, Eiler H. Inhibition of collagenase breakdown of equine corneas by tetanus antitoxin, equine serum and acetylcysteine. Vet Ophthalmol 2003;6(1):67–72.
13. Eaton JS, Hollingsworth SR, Holmberg BJ, et al. Effects of topically applied heterologous serum on reepithelialization rate of superficial chronic corneal epithelial defects in dogs. J Am Vet Med Assoc 2017;250(9):1014–22.
14. Okumura Y, Inomata T, Fujimoto K, et al. Biological effects of stored platelet-rich plasmaeye-drops in corneal wound healing. Br J Ophthalmol 2022;1–8.
15. Rushton J, Kammergruber E, Tichy A, et al. Effects of three blood derived products on equine corneal cells, an in vitro study. Equine Vet J 2018;50(3):356–62.
16. Hosny OH, Abd-Elkareem M, Ali MM, et al. Effect of autologous serum derived from advanced platelet-rich fibrin on the healing of experimentally-induced corneal ulcer in donkeys (equus asinus). J Adv Vet Res 2022;12(1):73–85.
17. Galera PD, Ribeiro CR, Sapp HL, et al. Proteomic analysis of equine amniotic membrane: characterization of proteins. Vet Ophthalmol 2015;18(3):198–209.
18. Lyons VN, Townsend WM, Moore GE, et al. Commercial amniotic membrane extract for treatment of corneal ulcers in adult horses. Equine Vet J 2021;53(6): 1268–76.
19. Boss CK, Gibson DJ, Schultz G, et al. Therapeutic effects of equine amniotic membrane suspension on corneal re-epithelialization and haze in a modified lagomorph ex vivo wound healing model. Vet Ophthalmol 2022;25(2):153–64.
20. Sherman AB, Gilger BC, Berglund AK, et al. Effect of bone marrow-derived mesenchymal stem cells and stem cell supernatant on equine corneal wound healing in vitro. Stem Cell Res Ther 2017;8(1):1–10.
21. Gilger BC, Michau TM, Salmon JH. Immune-mediated keratitis in horses: 19 cases (1998–2004). Vet Ophthalmol 2005;8(4):233–9.
22. Matthews A, Gilger B. Equine immune-mediated keratopathies. Equine Vet J 2010;42(S37):31–7.
23. Gilger BC, Stoppini R, Wilkie DA, et al. Treatment of immune-mediated keratitis in horses with episcleral silicone matrix cyclosporine delivery devices. Vet Ophthalmol 2014;17:23–30.
24. Almaliotis D, Koliakos G, Papakonstantinou E, et al. Mesenchymal stem cells improve healing of the cornea after alkali injury. Graefe's Arch Clin Exp Ophthalmol 2015;253(7):1121–35.
25. Cejka C, Holan V, Trosan P, et al. The favorable effect of mesenchymal stem cell treatment on the antioxidant protective mechanism in the corneal epithelium and renewal of corneal optical properties changed after alkali burns. Oxid Med Cell Longev 2016;2016:1–12.
26. Cejkova J, Trosan P, Cejka C, et al. Suppression of alkali-induced oxidative injury in the cornea by mesenchymal stem cells growing on nanofiber scaffolds and transferred onto the damaged corneal surface. Exp Eye Res 2013;116:312–23.
27. da Silva Meirelles L, Fontes AM, Covas DT, et al. Mechanisms involved in the therapeutic properties of mesenchymal stem cells. Cytokine Growth Factor Rev 2009; 20(5–6):419–27.

28. Gerding JC, Gilger BC. Prognosis and impact of equine recurrent uveitis. Equine Vet J 2016;48(3):290–8.
29. Deeg CA, Hauck SM, Amann B, et al. Equine recurrent uveitis - A spontaneous horse model of uveitis. Ophthalmic Res 2008;40(3–4):151–3.
30. Malalana F, Stylianides A, McGowan C. Equine recurrent uveitis: Human and equine perspectives. Vet J 2015;206(1):22–9.
31. Kol A, Wood JA, Carrade Holt DD, et al. Multiple intravenous injections of allogeneic equine mesenchymal stem cells do not induce a systemic inflammatory response but do alter lymphocyte subsets in healthy horses. Stem Cell Res Ther 2015;6(1):1–9.
32. Bastola P, Song L, Gilger BC, et al. Adeno-Associated Virus Mediated Gene Therapy for Corneal Diseases. Pharmaceutics 2020;12(8):767.
33. Miraldi Utz V, Coussa RG, Antaki F, et al. Gene therapy for RPE65-related retinal disease. Ophthalmic Genet 2018;39(6):671–7.
34. Patel U, Boucher M, de Léséleuc L, et al. Voretigene Neparvovec: An Emerging Gene Therapy for the Treatment of Inherited Blindness. 2018. In: CADTH Issues in Emerging Health Technologies. Ottawa (ON): Canadian Agency for Drugs and Technologies in Health; 2016, 169. Available at: https://www-ncbi-nlm-nih-gov.prox.lib.ncsu.edu/books/NBK538375/.
35. Moore KW, de Waal Malefyt R, Coffman RL, et al. Interleukin-10 and the interleukin-10 receptor. Annu Rev Immunol 2001;19:683.
36. Iyer SS and Cheng G. Role of interleukin 10 transcriptional regulation in inflammation and autoimmune disease, *Crit Rev Immunol*, 32 (1), 2012, 1-43.
37. Crabtree E, Uribe K, Smith SM, et al. Inhibition of experimental autoimmune uveitis by intravitreal AAV-Equine-IL10 gene therapy. PLoS One 2022;17(8):e0270972.
38. MacDonald ES, Barrett JG. The potential of mesenchymal stem cells to treat systemic inflammation in horses. Front Vet Sci 2020;6:507.

Use of Biologics and Stem Cells in the Treatment of Other Inflammatory Diseases in the Horse

Jennifer G. Barrett, PhD, DVM, DACVS, DACVSMR*,
Elizabeth S. MacDonald, BVMS, MS, DACVIM

KEYWORDS

- Mesenchymal stem cells • Endotoxemia • Recurrent airway obstruction
- Inflammatory bowel disease • Laminitis

KEY POINTS

- Mesenchymal stem cells (MSCs) modulate the immune system.
- MSCs are an exciting potential treatment of inflammatory conditions in the horse.
- More research is needed to determine the optimal cell type, source, preparation, route of delivery, dose, and schedule for treating horses.

MESENCHYMAL STEM CELLS MODULATE THE IMMUNE SYSTEM

De Schauwer and colleagues proposed that the definition of equine mesenchymal stem cells (MSCs) should be as follows: (1) the cells are plastic adherent, (2) they undergo trilineage differentiation (adipose, cartilage, and bone), and (3) they express CD29, CD44, and CD90 and not CD14, CD79α, or MHC-II.[1] Tissue sources of MSCs with these demonstrated properties include bone marrow, adipose, and umbilical cord blood.[2] In addition to their ability to differentiate, MSCs have powerful anti-inflammatory and immune-enhancing effects. In the authors' opinion, if immunologists had studied MSCs first, they likely would have been considered part of the immune system. MSCs produce a large number of cytokines, growth factors, chemokines, and immunomodulatory factors that influence the cells around them.[3] They play a role in increasing angiogenesis and inhibiting or inducing apoptosis.[4] MSCs are able to induce apoptosis of activated T cells, decrease T cell proliferation, and alter T cell phenotype.[5] MSCs also induce the expansion of regulatory T cells.[6] MSCs

Marion duPont Scott Equine Medical Center, Virginia-Maryland College of Veterinary Medicine, Virginia Tech, Leesburg, VA, USA
* Corresponding author.
E-mail address: jgbarrett@vt.edu

Vet Clin Equine 39 (2023) 553–563
https://doi.org/10.1016/j.cveq.2023.07.004 vetequine.theclinics.com
0749-0739/23/

exhibit these functions even when there is no direct cell contact,[7] highlighting the importance of the secretion of soluble factors and release of extracellular vesicles. In the correct environment, MSCs are activated to express several inhibitory factors including nitric oxide, indoleamine 2,3-dioxygenase (IDO), interleukin (IL)-10, transforming growth factor–β (TGF-β), tumor necrosis factor- (TNF) stimulated gene-6 (TSG-6), and prostaglandin E2 (PGE2) as well as surface molecules intercellular adhesion molecule 1 (ICAM-1) and vascular cell adhesion molecule (VCAM) and several growth factors including epidermal growth factor (EGF), fibroblast growth factors (FGF), platelet-derived growth factor (PDGF), vascular endothelial growth factor (VEGF), and stromal cell-derived factor 1 (SDF-1).[3,8,9]

More recently, investigations have turned toward MSC exosomes and their role in immunomodulation in response to injury. Exosomes are a class of extracellular vesicle that are purposely packaged to aid in cell–cell signaling.[10] These membrane-bound bodies can be released locally and taken up by neighboring cells, or released into circulation for a more systemic effect. Being membrane-bound, their contents are protected from proteases and endonucleases (which break down RNA signaling molecules). A multitude of signaling molecules is carried by exosomes, including cytokines and microRNAs.[10] MSC exosomes are being investigated as a therapy without the use of MSCs in the patient, perhaps facilitating regulatory clearance by the US Food and Drug Administration, and perhaps avoiding immune clearance over time. Equine exosomes can be isolated and studied similar to other species, and some of the therapeutic effects demonstrated in research studies using MSCs are likely due to exosomes.[11]

MSCs have also been shown to directly rescue cells that are damaged via mitochondrial transfer from the MSC to the damaged cell.[2] A relevant example of this is mitochondrial transfer to damaged leukocytes showed a preference for rescuing CD4+ T cells, rather than CD8+ T cells or CD19+ B cells.[12] In equine orthopedic research, MSCs were shown to donate mitochondria to damaged chondrocytes.[13] This mechanism requires the use of MSCs rather than cell-free exosomes for therapy; thus, MSC therapy may prove more beneficial for certain conditions.

HOW MESENCHYMAL STEM CELLS MODULATE THE IMMUNE SYSTEM

There is strong evidence that stem cells need to be primed or "licensed" to become effective at immunomodulation.[4] Exposure to proinflammatory molecules such as interferon gamma (IFN-γ), tumor necrosis factor alpha (TNF-α), IL-1, and lipopolysaccharide (LPS) activates MSCs into an anti-inflammatory state and assists homing of MSCs to sites of inflammation where they release growth factors, cytokines, and extracellular vesicles to promote healing and repair.[3,14] MSC homing to the site of injury is aided by VCAM-1 and E selectin activated by injured endothelial cells.[8] After priming human MSCs with IFN-γ and TNF-α, they were more effective at inhibiting T cell proliferation.[15] Priming of equine MSCs with TNF-α or IFN-γ induced significant upregulation of VCAM-1, IDO, inducible nitric oxide synthase (iNOS), and IL-6.[16] Primed equine MSCs decrease production of TNF-α and IFN-γ while showing increased production of PGE_2 and IL-6.[17] Three-dimensional culture of MSCs has also been shown to induce a more anti-inflammatory phenotype, including upregulation of IL-10 without the use of inflammatory mediators that may contaminate the cell suspension.[18] In contrast, quiescent equine MSCs derived from multiple sources (bone marrow, adipose tissue, and umbilical cord tissue) do not alter lymphocyte proliferation or secrete IL-6 or PGE_2 but did secrete TGF-β.[17] These findings further support the fact that MSCs must be exposed to inflammatory mediators to exhibit their immunosuppressive abilities and that careful optimization of MSC preparation is critical for their therapeutic potential.

Most research using horses does not address the need for priming MSCs before use. Phenotype, differentiation potential, and gene expression are also altered by how much the cells are expanded in cell culture.[19,20] In vivo studies in the horse vary as to how many times MSCs have doubled in culture before therapeutic use, which is the in vitro process of cellular aging. Another potential issue with published studies is that growing MSCs in standard fetal bovine serum (FBS) media induces immunogenicity in horses, and the antigens from FBS remain in MSCs unless the cells are grown for 24 hours in FBS-free culture media.[21] Growth in FBS-containing media also reduced MSC efficacy in an LPS synovitis model in horses.[22] The majority of published in vivo equine studies use MSCs grown in FBS-containing media without a washout period of growth in culture to reduce or remove the offending antigens.[23–25] Unless research studies using potentially aged, unprimed MSCs, contaminated with FBS, are repeated, we cannot truly understand the therapeutic potential of MSCs in horses. Going forward, it is critical for researchers to notice these factors in their studies, and for clinicians to be aware of the high degree of influence these issues have on the therapeutic potential of MSCs.

Another consideration for MSCs is whether they are autologous (from the patient themselves) or allogeneic (from a donor). In terms of using allogeneic sources, MSCs generally express low concentrations of major histocompatibility complex-I and do not express major histocompatibility complex-II (MHC-II),[26] which contributes to a potential lack of immunogenicity. However, priming MSCs to activate their anti-inflammatory phenotype can upregulate MHC-II.[27]

MSCs act through secretion of soluble factors (or exosomes) or direct cell-to-cell contact to modulate T cells, NK cells, B cells, and dendritic cells. MSCs induce apoptosis of activated T cells, induce cell cycle arrest, decrease T cell proliferation, and alter T cell phenotype. They target CD4+ and CD8+ T cell subsets equally.[28] Equine bone marrow-derived MSCs have been shown to exhibit a dose-dependent immunosuppression of T cell subsets.[29] Furthermore, both autologous and allogeneic MSCs showed equivalent degrees of suppression of T cell proliferation.[30] MSCs alter NK cell phenotype and suppress cytokine-induced proliferation of NK cells.[31] MSCs also promote the survival and inhibit the proliferation and maturation of B cells by arresting them in the G_0/G_1 phase of the cell cycle.[32] MSCs can also modulate dendritic cell maturation, differentiation, and function.[33] In mice, it has been suggested that MSCs decrease the proliferation of B cells,[4] and this has also been demonstrated in an in vitro equine study.[34]

In human medicine, the immunomodulatory, cell rescue, and anti-inflammatory properties have been in sharper focus than in equines.[35] Primed anti-inflammatory MSCs harbor great potential for the treatment of endotoxemia, recurrent airway obstruction/equine asthma, inflammatory bowel diseases (IBDs) and laminitis in horses but much research remains to optimize and study their potential in these clinical areas. Going forward, it is critical for researchers to avoid using FBS-tainted cells, to optimize the anti-inflammatory phenotype and age of MSCs before use, and to determine whether autologous or allogeneic cells and which tissue source of MSCs is optimal for the condition they are studying.

ENDOTOXEMIA IN THE HORSE

Colic remains the leading cause of death in the adult horse, and reports show that mortality is very closely related to the degree of endotoxemia.[36,37] Of the adult horses that present to referral hospitals for colic, 30% to 40% have detectable endotoxin in their circulation.[38] Higher concentrations of endotoxin at admission and intraoperatively have been associated with increased mortality.[39] Although the gastrointestinal tract is the most common source of endotoxin, and strangulating or obstructive lesions are the most common cause, endotoxemia can be caused by any gram-negative bacterial infection that may occur in colitis, peritonitis, pleuropneumonia, and metritis. Of the foals that present for septicemia, up to 50% have detectable circulating endotoxin.[40]

To date, there is no single effective treatment of endotoxemia in horses. The goal of therapy is to reduce or prevent the movement of endotoxin into circulation, neutralize circulating endotoxin, reduce interaction with inflammatory cells, prevent the synthesis of proinflammatory mediators, and supportive care. There are limited treatment options available, such as nonsteroidal anti-inflammatory drugs, intravenous fluids, hyperimmune plasma, polymyxin B, and dimethyl sulfoxide.[41,42] The long list of potential treatment options shows that there remains an unmet need for a safe and effective treatment of endotoxemia in the horse.

Mesenchymal Stem Cells Alleviate Endotoxemia in Rodent Models

A mouse model of endotoxemia show a systemic inflammatory response, alterations in lung structure and function, increased numbers of inflammatory cells in the lung, and pulmonary edema.[43] MSC treatment in this model resulted in amelioration of all of those symptoms, similar to normal mice.[43] Cecal ligation and puncture (CLP) is another model of inflammation, sepsis, and endotoxemia. After undergoing the CLP procedure, mice develop clinical signs associated with sepsis from the infection that is established within the peritoneal cavity and mimics the course of sepsis.[44] When mice subjected to CLP are treated with MSCs, they exhibit decreased production of plasma IL-6, IL-1β, and IL-10; had improved bacterial clearance; and reduced mortality by 50% compared with controls.[45] The potential benefit of MSC therapy for sepsis was documented in a preclinical meta-analysis showing that the overall odds of death in rodents with sepsis was reduced by treatment with MSCs.[46] Overall, there is strong evidence that MSCs may be beneficial in the treatment of endotoxemia in rodent models.

Mesenchymal Stem Cells Have Not Ameliorated Endotoxemia in Equine Studies

A randomized placebo-controlled in vivo study investigating the effect of allogeneic peripheral blood derived MSCs on endotoxemia did not ameliorate the clinical signs.[25] MSCs (that were grown using FBS media) were delivered intravenously to horses that were induced into endotoxemia with an intravenous infusion of LPS. The only parameter that improved was IL-1 levels in serum.[25] A smaller LPS pilot study using bone marrow-derived MSCs also failed to show improvement in the clinical signs of endotoxemia.[47] Given the lack of response in these studies, abandoning MSC therapy for endotoxemia may be tempting. However, optimizing the source and preparation of the cells, and repeating with a dose response trial may be worthwhile.

RECURRENT AIRWAY OBSTRUCTION IN THE HORSE

Recurrent airway obstruction (RAO) in horses is an inflammatory disease process similar to asthma characterized by excessive mucus production, neutrophil accumulation, bronchial hyperreactivity, and reversible bronchospasm. Hypersensitivity to inhaled molds and other organic dusts is thought to be the initiating cause with a prevalence from 2% to 80% depending on the inclusion criteria of the study.[48] The underlying immunologic mechanisms that lead to pulmonary inflammation have not been fully described at this time. In an unaffected horse, any possible stimulus (molds or dust) that enters the airway is cleared by the immune system. In affected horses, this stimulus activates lymphocytes, leading to neutrophil recruitment and inflammation within the airway. There is an influx of neutrophils into the airways with an increase in CD4+ T cells in bronchial alveolar lavage fluid.[49] Treatment of all species is limited to environmental management, anti-inflammatory therapy, and bronchodilator therapy. For horses, the use of corticosteroids, the mainstay of treatment, may be contraindicated in some patients. Inhaled corticosteroids, which reduce the risk of complications, are now available as well.

Mesenchymal Stem Cells Alleviate Asthma Symptoms in Mice

RAO is similar to asthma seen in humans and cats but the disease process varies in that asthma is dominated by an influx of eosinophils rather than of neutrophils. Experimental studies using murine models of ovalbumin-induced asthma have shown that stem cells may be beneficial for managing the disease process. After one injection of human stem cells, there was a significant decrease in the presence of eosinophils in bronchial alveolar lavage fluid; a significant reduction in IL-5, IL-13, and IFN-γ; and a decrease in circulating IgE concentrations.[50] An improvement was shown histologically as well with the treated mice exhibiting a decrease in airway inflammation, goblet cell hyperplasia, epithelial cell lining thickening, and collagen deposition. Similar results were shown in a ragweed-induced murine model of asthma.[51] MSCs have shown benefits when administered either by intravenously or by intratracheal delivery. Immunomodulatory effects were more predominant after intravenous injection while intratracheal delivery resulted in a more reparative mechanism in rodent models.[52]

Mesenchymal Stem Cells Ameliorate Recurrent Airway Obstruction in Horses

An in vitro study looking at the response of LPS stimulated equine alveolar macrophages after exposure to conditioned medium and microvesicles (exosomes) from amniotic-derived MSCs showed there was a significant decrease in TNF-α production in the treated group compared with controls.[53] These findings show that the amniotic MSC derivatives are capable of altering the alveolar macrophages cytokine release and may be able to play a role in treating inflammatory diseases affecting the equine lung.

For equine RAO, adipose-derived autologous MSCs improved symptoms in a controlled clinical trial of equine severe asthma.[23] Horses that were treated with intrabronchial MSCs had improved short-term clinical scores, positive long-term clinical effects, and decreased expression of IL-17, IL-1β, IL-4, and TNFα. In a different approach, intratracheal bone marrow mononuclear cells were compared with dexamethasone treatment in a controlled trial in horses with naturally occurring RAO. Both treatments improved clinical signs and decreased neutrophils and increased macrophages in lavage fluid on day 7 and 14.[54] Although MSCs may be beneficial in the treatment of RAO, the timing of their administration may play a role in response to treatment. The number of doses and follow-up treatment need to be investigated.

GASTROINTESTINAL SYSTEM AND MESENCHYMAL STEM CELLS

There are 5 conditions of the gastrointestinal system that have shown promise in rodent models and canine or human clinical trials for treatment by MSCs: (1) IBD,[55] (2) peritonitis,[56] (3) colitis,[57,58] (4) gastric ulceration,[59] and (5) adhesion prevention.[60]

Mesenchymal Stem Cells Improve Clinical Signs of Inflammatory Bowel Disease and Colitis in Other Species

IBD is a broad term used to describe several small and large intestinal disorders in animals. In small animals and horses, infiltration of the GI submucosa and mucosa with eosinophils, plasma cells, lymphocytes, basophils, or macrophages causes IBD.[61] The cause is often unknown and the type of cell that infiltrates the mucosa and submucosa can affect prognosis. In humans, IBD represents a specific disease process such as ulcerative colitis (the colon only is affected) or Crohn disease (any part of the gastrointestinal tract is affected).[62] The clinical signs include diarrhea, weight loss, dependent edema, and lethargy and are often associated with protein-losing enteropathy and malabsorption. The pathogenesis of IBD was thought to be inflammation mediated by the acquired immune system with an imbalance between the Th1 cells and proinflammatory cytokines overcoming the control mechanisms. An alternative theory proposes that it could be a primary failure of regulatory lymphocytes and cytokines to control inflammation.[63] The current goals of treatment of humans are directed at relieving inflammation and treating signs and symptoms.[64] The only treatment available for horses at this time is corticosteroid therapy and the response is often poor.[65] Stem cells could prove to be a good alternative.[55,62] Initial phase one trials of bone marrow derived stem cells for the treatment of refractory Crohn disease in humans have produced mixed results. Some patients have shown improvement by reduction in their clinical assessment score, improvement in the mucosa on endoscopy, and reduction of inflammation and presence of cytokines on biopsy.[62]

Mesenchymal Stem Cells Improve Gastric Ulcer Healing and Reduce Adhesion Formation in Mice

Murine models have also shown other benefits of stem cells in the gastrointestinal system. Stem cells can accelerate gastric ulcer healing by homing to the site of injury. Labeled stem cells have been found only in the injured gastric mucosa and not in the normal mucosa.[59] The route of administration for the treatment of gastrointestinal disease is important. Mice with induced colitis that received intravenous stem cells showed a significant reduction in clinical and histopathologic severity when compared with mice that received stems cells intraperitoneal stem cells.[66] Stem cells have also shown benefits when injected intravenously to attenuate peritoneal adhesions in experimentally induced lesions in mice.[60] If systemic treatment with MSCs adequately attenuates inflammation after intestinal insult and thereby reduces the risk of adhesions in horses, a very practical allogeneic MSC therapy may be possible.

MESENCHYMAL STEM CELL TREATMENT OF LAMINITIS IN THE HORSE

Laminitis, a devastating inflammatory condition of the hoof, may also benefit from MSC therapy. Horses with bilateral laminitis were treated in one limb with adipose-derived MSCs, and saline control in the opposite limb. MSC-treated limbs had improved hoof growth and vascular perfusion when compared with control.[67] Epidermal progenitor stem cells have been successfully cultured from horses and may be useful to treat laminitis in the future.[68,69] MSC delivery to the hoof has been well-studied, and arterial perfusion is a viable delivery of high doses of MSCs to the vasculature of the hoof.[70] The difficulty in assessing MSC therapy to treat laminitis is the variability of case presentations in terms of severity and chronicity. Once an optimal anti-inflammatory MSC therapy is developed, testing it in a laminitis model would be helpful to determine optimum timing, frequency, and duration of treatment of this disease.

SUMMARY

There is a huge potential for stem cells to treat a wide range of conditions in the horse. The therapeutic potential is attributed to the unique properties of the MSC that target damaged tissues, inhibit the immune and inflammatory response, and facilitate repair. Several researches are needed to test the efficacy and safety of these novel treatments in equines. This will require properly constructed clinical trials that are often challenging to perform and are currently lacking. The challenges moving forward include identifying if there is an ideal MSC donor and ensure that they are screened for any potential systemic diseases. The ideal timing of injection needs to be identified so that the environment may be able to promote the best activity of MSCs but not so advanced that the tissues cannot be repaired or recovered. MSC have multiple pathways through which they achieve their immune suppression and anti-inflammatory roles of which the mechanisms have not all been determined at this time. Identifying the best way to activate MSCs to get the most therapeutic potential will be essential. Furthermore, it will also be critical to optimize culture conditions to remove FBS contamination and to ensure the age of the MSCs is consistent with optimal efficacy.

CLINICS CARE POINTS

- Avoid using MSCs grown in fetal bovine serum media.
- Consider age of donor and how many times the MSCs have been dividing in cell culture.

DISCLOSURE

No conflicts of interest.

REFERENCES

1. De Schauwer C, Meyer E, Van de Walle GR, et al. Markers of stemness in equine mesenchymal stem cells: a plea for uniformity. Theriogenology 2011;75:1431–43.
2. Spees JL, Lee RH, Gregory CA. Mechanisms of mesenchymal stem/stromal cell function. Stem Cell Res Ther 2016;7:125.
3. Shi Y, Su J, Roberts AI, et al. How mesenchymal stem cells interact with tissue immune responses. Trends Immunol 2012;33:136–43.
4. Singer NG, Caplan AI. Mesenchymal stem cells: mechanisms of inflammation. Annu Rev Pathol 2011;6:457–78.
5. Peroni JF, Borjesson DL. Anti-inflammatory and immunomodulatory activities of stem cells. Vet Clin N Am Equine Pract 2011;27:351–62.
6. Siegel G, Schafer R, Dazzi F. The immunosuppressive properties of mesenchymal stem cells. Transplantation 2009;87:S45–9.
7. Lavoie JR, Rosu-Myles M. Uncovering the secretes of mesenchymal stem cells. Biochimie 2013;95:2212–21.
8. Meirelles Lda S, Fontes AM, Covas DT, et al. Mechanisms involved in the therapeutic properties of mesenchymal stem cells. Cytokine Growth Factor Rev 2009;20:419–27.
9. Crisostomo PR, Wang Y, Markel TA, et al. Human mesenchymal stem cells stimulated by TNF-alpha, LPS, or hypoxia produce growth factors by an NF kappa B- but not JNK-dependent mechanism. Am J Physiol Cell Physiol 2008;294:C675–82.

10. Capomaccio S, Cappelli K, Bazzucchi C, et al. Equine Adipose-Derived Mesenchymal Stromal Cells Release Extracellular Vesicles Enclosing Different Subsets of Small RNAs. Stem Cell Int 2019;4957806.
11. Klymiuk MC, Balz N, Elashry MI, et al. Exosomes isolation and identification from equine mesenchymal stem cells. BMC Vet Res 2019;15(42).
12. Court AC, Le-Gatt A, Luz-Crawford P, et al. Mitochondrial transfer from MSCs to T cells induces Treg differentiation and restricts inflammatory response. EMBO Rep 2020;21:e48052.
13. Fahey M, Bennett M, Thomas M, et al. Mesenchymal stromal cells donate mitochondria to articular chondrocytes exposed to mitochondrial, environmental, and mechanical stress. Sci Rep 2022;12:21525.
14. Chen S, Sun F, Qian H, et al. Preconditioning and Engineering Strategies for Improving the Efficacy of Mesenchymal Stem Cell-Derived Exosomes in Cell-Free Therapy. Stem Cell Int 2022;1779346.
15. Cuerquis J, Romieu-Mourez R, François M, et al. Human mesenchymal stromal cells transiently increase cytokine production by activated T cells before suppressing T-cell proliferation: effect of interferon-γ and tumor necrosis factor-α stimulation. Cytotherapy 2014;16:191–202.
16. Barrachina L, Remacha AR, Romero A, et al. Priming Equine Bone Marrow-Derived Mesenchymal Stem Cells with Proinflammatory Cytokines: Implications in Immunomodulation-Immunogenicity Balance, Cell Viability, and Differentiation Potential. Stem Cell Dev 2017;26:15–24.
17. Carrade DD, Lame MW, Kent MS, et al. Comparative Analysis of the Immunomodulatory Properties of Equine Adult-Derived Mesenchymal Stem Cells. Cell Med 2012;4:1–11.
18. Bogers SH, Barrett JG. Three-Dimensional Culture of Equine Bone Marrow-Derived Mesenchymal Stem Cells Enhances Anti-Inflammatory Properties in a Donor-Dependent Manner. Stem Cell Dev 2022;31:777–86.
19. Wagner W, Horn P, Castoldi M, et al. Replicative senescence of mesenchymal stem cells: a continuous and organized process. PLoS One 2008;3:e2213.
20. Liu J, Ding Y, Liu Z, et al. Senescence in Mesenchymal Stem Cells: Functional Alterations, Molecular Mechanisms, and Rejuvenation Strategies. Front Cell Dev Biol 2020;8:258.
21. Joswig AJ, Mitchell A, Cummings KJ, et al. Repeated intra-articular injection of allogeneic mesenchymal stem cells causes an adverse response compared to autologous cells in the equine model. Stem Cell Res Ther 2017;8:42.
22. Rowland AL, Burns ME, Levine GJ, et al. Preparation Technique Affects Recipient Immune Targeting of Autologous Mesenchymal Stem Cells. Front Vet Sci 2021;8:724041.
23. Adamic N, Prpar Mihevc S, Blagus R, et al. Effect of intrabronchial administration of autologous adipose-derived mesenchymal stem cells on severe equine asthma. Stem Cell Res Ther 2022;13(23).
24. Ardanaz N, Vazquez FJ, Romero A, et al. Inflammatory response to the administration of mesenchymal stem cells in an equine experimental model: effect of autologous, and single and repeat doses of pooled allogeneic cells in healthy joints. BMC Vet Res 2016;12:65.
25. Taylor SD, Serpa PBS, Santos AP, et al. Effects of intravenous administration of peripheral blood-derived mesenchymal stromal cells after infusion of lipopolysaccharide in horses. J Vet Intern Med 2022;36:1491–501.

26. Wang S, Zhao RC. A Historical Overview and Concepts of Mesenchymal Stem Cells. In: Zhao RC, editor. Essentials of mesenchymal stem cell biology and its clinical translation. Dordrecht: Springer; 2013. p. 3–15.
27. Barrachina L, Remacha AR, Romero A, et al. Effect of inflammatory environment on equine bone marrow derived mesenchymal stem cells immunogenicity and immunomodulatory properties. Vet Immunol Immunopathol 2016;171:57–65.
28. Najar M, Raicevic G, Boufker HI, et al. Mesenchymal stromal cells use PGE2 to modulate activation and proliferation of lymphocyte subsets: Combined comparison of adipose tissue, Wharton's Jelly and bone marrow sources. Cell Immunol 2010;264:171–9.
29. Ranera B, Antczak D, Miller D, et al. Donor-derived equine mesenchymal stem cells suppress proliferation of mismatched lymphocytes. Equine Vet J 2016;48: 253–60.
30. Colbath AC, Dow SW, Phillips JN, et al. Autologous and Allogeneic Equine Mesenchymal Stem Cells Exhibit Equivalent Immunomodulatory Properties In Vitro. Stem Cell Dev 2017;26:503–11.
31. Rasmusson I, Le Blanc K, Sundberg B, et al. Mesenchymal stem cells stimulate antibody secretion in human B cells. Scand J Immunol 2007;65:336–43.
32. Tabera S, Perez-Simon JA, Diez-Campelo M, et al. The effect of mesenchymal stem cells on the viability, proliferation and differentiation of B-lymphocytes. Haematologica 2008;93:1301–9.
33. Zhang B, Liu R, Shi D, et al. Mesenchymal stem cells induce mature dendritic cells into a novel Jagged-2-dependent regulatory dendritic cell population. Blood 2009;113:46–57.
34. Cequier A, Romero A, Vazquez FJ, et al. Equine Mesenchymal Stem Cells Influence the Proliferative Response of Lymphocytes: Effect of Inflammation, Differentiation and MHC-Compatibility. Animals (Basel) 2022;12.
35. Borjesson DL, Peroni JF. The regenerative medicine laboratory: facilitating stem cell therapy for equine disease. Clin Lab Med 2011;31:109–23.
36. Thoefner MB, Ersboll AK, Jensen AL, et al. Factor analysis of the interrelationships between clinical variables in horses with colic. Prev Vet Med 2001;48: 201–14.
37. Tinker MK, White NA, Lessard P, et al. Prospective study of equine colic incidence and mortality. Equine Vet J 1997;29:448–53.
38. Senior JM, Proudman CJ, Leuwer M, et al. Plasma endotoxin in horses presented to an equine referral hospital: correlation to selected clinical parameters and outcomes. Equine Vet J 2011;43:585–91.
39. Steverink PJ, Salden HJ, Sturk A, et al. Laboratory and clinical evaluation of a chromogenic endotoxin assay for horses with acute intestinal disorders. Vet Q 1994;16:117–21.
40. Barton MH. Endotoxemia. In: Sprayberry K, Robinson N, editors. Robinson's current therapy in equine medicine. . St. Louis, Missouri: Elsevier; 2003. p. 104–8.
41. Moore JN, Barton MH, Treatment of endotoxemia. Vet Clin N Am Equine Pract 2003;19:681–95.
42. Sykes BW, Furr MO. Equine endotoxaemia–a state-of-the-art review of therapy. Aust Vet J 2005;83:45–50.
43. Xu J, Woods CR, Mora AL, et al. Prevention of endotoxin-induced systemic response by bone marrow-derived mesenchymal stem cells in mice. Am J Physiol Lung Cell Mol Physiol 2007;293:L131–41.
44. Buras JA, Holzmann B, Sitkovsky M. Animal models of sepsis: setting the stage. Nat Rev Drug Discov 2005;4:854–65.

45. Mei SH, Haitsma JJ, Dos Santos CC, et al. Mesenchymal stem cells reduce inflammation while enhancing bacterial clearance and improving survival in sepsis. Am J Respir Crit Care Med 2010;182:1047–57.
46. Lalu MM, Sullivan KJ, Mei SH, et al. Evaluating mesenchymal stem cell therapy for sepsis with preclinical meta-analyses prior to initiating a first-in-human trial. Elife 2016;5.
47. Kilcoyne I, Nieto JE, Watson JL, et al. Do allogeneic bone marrow derived mesenchymal stem cells diminish the inflammatory response to lipopolysaccharide infusion in horses? A pilot study. Vet Immunol Immunopathol 2021. https://doi.org/10.1016/j.vetimm.2020.110146.
48. Leguillette R. Recurrent airway obstruction–heaves. Vet Clin N Am Equine Pract 2003;19:63–86, vi.
49. Pirie RS. Recurrent airway obstruction: a review. Equine Vet J 2014;46:276–88.
50. Bonfield TL, Koloze M, Lennon DP, et al. Human mesenchymal stem cells suppress chronic airway inflammation in the murine ovalbumin asthma model. Am J Physiol Lung Cell Mol Physiol 2010;299:L760–70.
51. Nemeth K, Keane-Myers A, Brown JM, et al. Bone marrow stromal cells use TGF-beta to suppress allergic responses in a mouse model of ragweed-induced asthma. Proc Natl Acad Sci U S A 2010;107:5652–7.
52. Antunes MA, Lapa ESJR, Rocco PR. Mesenchymal stromal cell therapy in COPD: from bench to bedside. Int J Chronic Obstr Pulm Dis 2017;12:3017–27.
53. Zucca E, Corsini E, Galbiati V, et al. Evaluation of amniotic mesenchymal cell derivatives on cytokine production in equine alveolar macrophages: an in vitro approach to lung inflammation. Stem Cell Res Ther 2016;7:137.
54. Barussi FC, Bastos FZ, Leite LM, et al. Intratracheal therapy with autologous bone marrow-derived mononuclear cells reduces airway inflammation in horses with recurrent airway obstruction. Respir Physiol Neurobiol 2016;232:35–42.
55. Saadh MJ, Mikhailova MV, Rasoolzadegan S, et al. Therapeutic potential of mesenchymal stem/stromal cells (MSCs)-based cell therapy for inflammatory bowel diseases (IBD) therapy. Eur J Med Res 2023;28:47.
56. Kato T, Murata A, Ishida H, et al. Interleukin 10 reduces mortality from severe peritonitis in mice. Antimicrob Agents Chemother 1995;39:1336–40.
57. Gonzalez-Rey E, Anderson P, Gonzalez MA, et al. Human adult stem cells derived from adipose tissue protect against experimental colitis and sepsis. Gut 2009;58:929–39.
58. Gonzalez MA, Gonzalez-Rey E, Rico L, et al. Adipose-derived mesenchymal stem cells alleviate experimental colitis by inhibiting inflammatory and autoimmune responses. Gastroenterology 2009;136:978–89.
59. Chang Q, Yan L, Wang CZ, et al. In vivo transplantation of bone marrow mesenchymal stem cells accelerates repair of injured gastric mucosa in rats. Chin Med J (Engl) 2012;125:1169–74.
60. Wang N, Shao Y, Mei Y, et al. Novel mechanism for mesenchymal stem cells in attenuating peritoneal adhesion: accumulating in the lung and secreting tumor necrosis factor alpha-stimulating gene-6. Stem Cell Res Ther 2012;3:51.
61. Schumacher J, Edwards JF, Cohen ND. Chronic idiopathic inflammatory bowel diseases of the horse. J Vet Intern Med 2000;14:258–65.
62. Duijvestein M, Vos AC, Roelofs H, et al. Autologous bone marrow-derived mesenchymal stromal cell treatment for refractory luminal Crohn's disease: results of a phase I study. Gut 2010;59:1662–9.
63. Strober W, Fuss IJ. Pro-Inflammatory Cytokines in the Pathogenesis of IBD. Gastroenterology 2011;140:1756–67.

64. Panes J, Ordas I, Ricart E. Stem cell treatment for Crohn's disease. Expert Rev Clin Immunol 2010;6:597–605.
65. Barr BS. Infiltrative intestinal disease. Vet Clin N Am Equine Pract 2006;22:e1–7.
66. Goncalves Fda C, Schneider N, Pinto FO, et al. Intravenous vs intraperitoneal mesenchymal stem cells administration: what is the best route for treating experimental colitis? World J Gastroenterol 2014;20:18228–39.
67. Oliveira APL, Paz CFR, Lima MPA, et al. Radiographic, Venographic and Hoof Growth Evaluations in Equine Forelimbs with Chronic Laminitis Treated or Not with Mesenquimal Stem Cells Derived from Adipose Tissue. Cytotherapy 2021;23:31–2.
68. da Silva LL, Silveira MD, da Costa Garcia CAS, et al. Coronary corium, a new source of equine mesenchymal stromal cells. Vet Res Commun 2020;44:41–9.
69. Marycz K, Pielok A, Kornicka-Garbowska K. Equine Hoof Stem Progenitor Cells (HPC) CD29 +/Nestin +/K15 + - a Novel Dermal/epidermal Stem Cell Population With a Potential Critical Role for Laminitis Treatment. Stem Cell Rev Rep 2021;17:1478–85.
70. Trela JM, Spriet M, Padgett KA, et al. Scintigraphic comparison of intra-arterial injection and distal intravenous regional limb perfusion for administration of mesenchymal stem cells to the equine foot. Equine Vet J 2014;46:479–83.

Antimicrobial Properties of Equine Stromal Cells and Platelets and Future Directions

Lynn M. Pezzanite, DVM, MS, PhD, DACVS-LA[a,*], Lyndah Chow, PhD[a],
Steven W. Dow, DVM, PhD, DACVIM[a,b],
Laurie R. Goodrich, DVM, MS, PhD, DACVS[a],
Jessica M. Gilbertie, DVM, MS, PhD[c],
Lauren V. Schnabel, DVM, PhD, DACVS, DACVSMR[d,e,*]

KEYWORDS

• Horse • Antimicrobial • Regenerative • Biologic • Therapies
• Mesenchymal stromal cells • Platelets

KEY POINTS

- Both equine mesenchymal stromal cells (MSCs) and platelets exert potent antimicrobial and immunomodulatory effects through the secretion of antimicrobial peptides and cytokines that alter the host immune response, making them attractive as an adjunctive therapy in the treatment of bacterial infections.
- Antimicrobial effects of MSCs may be upregulated by priming with exposure to toll and nod-like receptors that are typically present in inflammation and infection prior to clinical application.
- Further investigation of MSC extracellular vesicle-based therapies is indicated to harness the paracrine influence of MSCs while eliminating regulatory concerns regarding the use of cell-based therapies and practical issues with the implementation of allogeneic products.
- Pooled allogeneic platelet lysate products are recommended for the treatment of bacterial infections and particularly biofilm-based infections and are markedly different in manufacturing technique and composition compared to traditional autologous platelet products such as platelet-rich plasma (PRP).
- While acellular in nature, pooled allogeneic platelet lysate products must still be carefully processed to avoid potential immunogenicity and donors must be screened to avoid potential transmission of infectious diseases.

---

[a] Department of Clinical Sciences, College of Veterinary Medicine and Biomedical Sciences, Colorado State University, Fort Collins, CO, USA; [b] Department of Microbiology, Immunology and Pathology, College of Veterinary Medicine and Biomedical Sciences, Colorado State University, Fort Collins, CO, USA; [c] Department of Microbiology and Immunology, Edward Via College of Osteopathic Medicine, Blacksburg, VA, USA; [d] Department of Clinical Sciences, College of Veterinary Medicine and Biomedical Sciences, North Carolina State University, Raleigh, NC, USA; [e] Comparative Medicine Institute, North Carolina State University, Raleigh, NC, USA
* Corresponding authors.
E-mail addresses: lynn.pezzanite@colostate.edu (L.M.P.); lvschnab@ncsu.edu (L.V.S.)

Vet Clin Equine 39 (2023) 565–578
https://doi.org/10.1016/j.cveq.2023.06.005 vetequine.theclinics.com

SUMMARY

Increasing antimicrobial resistance in veterinary practice has driven the investigation of novel therapeutic strategies including regenerative and biologic therapies to treat bacterial infection. Integration of biological approaches such as platelet lysate and mesenchymal stromal cell (MSC) therapy may represent adjunctive treatment strategies for bacterial infections that minimize systemic side effects and local tissue toxicity associated with traditional antibiotics and that are not subject to antibiotic resistance. In this review, we will discuss mechanisms by which biological therapies exert antimicrobial effects, as well as potential applications and challenges in clinical implementation in equine practice.

EVIDENCE FOR ANTIMICROBIAL PROPERTIES OF EQUINE MESENCHYMAL STROMAL CELLS

Mesenchymal stromal cells (MSC) from multiple tissue sources exert potent antibacterial and immunomodulatory activities, rendering them attractive as potential treatments for a number of diverse conditions in equine practice including systemic inflammation, orthopedic and ophthalmic disease, wound healing, and more recently, bacterial infection.[1–11] Evidence supporting mechanisms by which MSC from multiple veterinary species (equine, canine, bovine) exert an antimicrobial effect through the secretion of bioactive factors and indirectly through recruitment and activation of the patient's innate immune cells and interact with antibiotics has been recently reviewed[12] and are illustrated in **Fig. 1**.

Mechanisms of constitutive antimicrobial action of equine MSCs specifically were initially investigated *in vitro* using peripheral blood-derived equine MSCs.[3,12] Harman and colleagues[3] (2017) first demonstrated that both MSC and MSC conditioned media (MSC-CM) inhibited the growth of both Gram positive and negative bacteria (*S. aureus* and *E. coli*) through membrane depolarization. They further identified four antimicrobial peptides (AMP) in equine MSC-CM, namely cathelicidin, elafin, lipocalin 2, and cystatin C, and demonstrated that blocking AMP activity using AMP-specific antibodies diminished the observed antimicrobial effect.[3] The same group of investigators confirmed these findings in a second study, where MSC-CM was shown to inhibit bacterial growth against a broader range of bacterial species tested (*P. aeruginosa, A. viridanns, A. baumannii, S. epidermis, S. aureus*), and were further demonstrated to secrete cysteine proteases that contributed to the destabilization of methicillin resistant *S. aureus* biofilms, which also enhanced the efficacy of antibiotic co-administration.[12] This observed effect (ie, that MSC administration results in additive or even synergistic reduction in quantitative bacterial counts has been corroborated by reports in other species and *in vivo* in horses as well,[10,13] providing further evidence to support the use of MSC and its secretome as complementary therapies in the treatment of multi-drug resistant or biofilm infections that may be otherwise recalcitrant to treatment.

METHODS TO ENHANCE ANTIMICROBIAL PROPERTIES OF MESENCHYMAL STROMAL CELLS

Mounting interest in the application of cell-based therapies in the treatment of infection has prompted further investigation of methods to enhance and optimize their antibacterial activity.[2,9,10,14] Techniques evaluated specifically using equine tissues have included the comparison of initial MSC tissue source, serum source in culture media, and priming or 'licensing' techniques to enhance antimicrobial activity prior to *in vivo* activation.

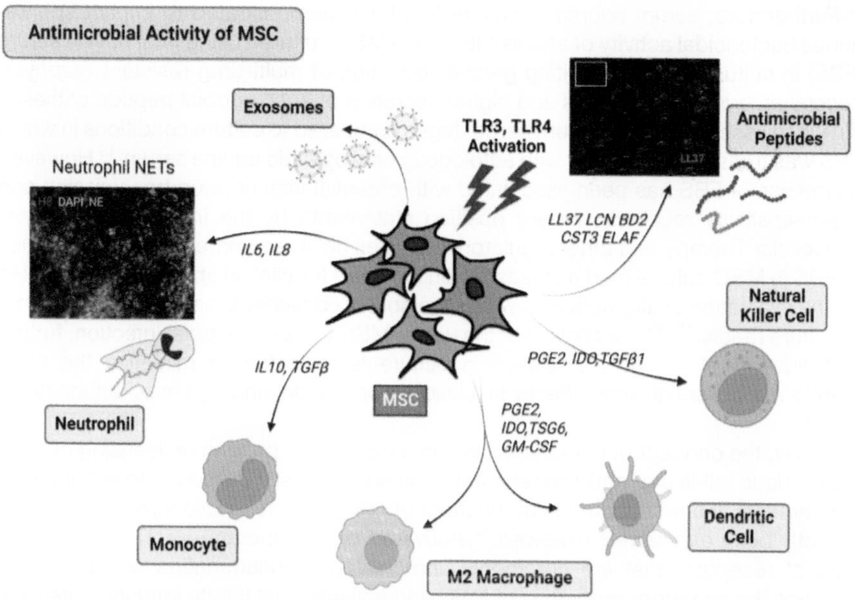

Fig. 1. *Immune mechanisms for antimicrobial properties of MSC against biofilms.* Direct antimicrobial activity of MSC via secreted factors including antimicrobial peptides and indirect immunomodulatory activity of MSC are illustrated. Directly, cationic antimicrobial peptides (eg, cathelicidin, lipocalin-2, ß-defensin 2), induce damage to bacterial membranes or alter bacterial function either directly or indirectly. Indirectly, MSC activate host immune cells, modulate local inflammation, and induce angiogenesis and fibrogenesis, targeting several different cell types including T cells, macrophages, neutrophils, and dendritic cells. This activity is primarily mediated by the up-regulation or inhibition of immunomodulatory cytokines and chemokines that in turn augment the immune system either to a pro-inflammatory or an anti-inflammatory state.

While equine MSC sourced from multiple different tissues (eg, peripheral blood, bone marrow, adipose, endometrium, umbilical cord) have demonstrated constitutive antimicrobial activity, few reports exist providing direct comparisons of functionality regarding their capacity for immune modulation or specifically for antimicrobial action. Cortes-Araya and colleagues.[2] provided an initial evaluation of the relative activity of equine MSC from three tissue sources (endometrium, bone marrow, and adipose). Interestingly, while MSC-CM from all sources inhibited the growth of planktonic *E. coli*, this effect was considered more prominent when using adipose or endometrium-derived tissues compared to bone marrow.[2] Production of antimicrobial peptide lipocalin-2 was also more pronounced in endometrium-derived cell cultures compared to the other two tissue sources. Finally, MSC from all sources were demonstrated to express immunomodulatory cytokines and markers TLR-4, chemokine ligand-5, monocyte chemoattractant protein-1, and interleukin-6 and 8 at detectable levels, although adipose-derived MSCs were not found to express macrophage marker colony-stimulating factor 1 receptor, which may to some degree impact different tissue sources' bearing on the induction of the innate immune system. A more comprehensive comparison of MSC derived from different tissue sources for bactericidal activity against both Gram-positive and negative bacterial cultures and biofilms is indicated to guide best practices in the clinical use of MSC for the purpose of infection control.

Furthermore, serum source in culture has been demonstrated to impact spontaneous bactericidal activity of equine MSC, with MSC cultured using fetal bovine serum (FBS) in culture media exhibiting greater reduction of multi-drug resistant *Staphylococcus aureus* colony counts and higher secretion of antimicrobial peptide cathelicidin when assessed at low serum percentages compared to culture conditions in which FBS was transiently replaced with autologous or allogeneic equine serum.[15] However, as the use of FBS has been associated with potential viral or prion transmission and hypersensitivity reactions, recent position statements by the International Society for Cellular Therapy and other regulatory agencies have recommended the avoidance of FBS in MSC culture media at least when intended for clinical application and called for the evaluation of alternatives towards the goal of consensus in serum replacements in culture media.[16–19] the context of the use of MSC to treat bacterial infection, further investigation of serum alternatives in culture is indicated to minimize the afore mentioned potential side effects in clinical application and optimize antibacterial effect.

Finally, the concept of immune activation, also termed priming or licensing of MSC with various toll-like or nod-like receptor agonists, has been proposed to enhance the antibacterial and immunomodulatory effect of MSC prior to *in vivo* injection, and has recently been extensively reviewed.[14] Activated cellular therapy (ACT) takes advantage of receptors that are commonly upregulated in inflammation or infection to enhance the migratory properties of MSC and activate host innate immune defenses. Evidence for enhanced efficacy with these techniques has been generated *in vitro* and in mouse models of biofilm infection,[9,13,20–23] indicating greater reduction in both planktonic and biofilm cultures and enhanced resolution of MRSA biofilms in mesh implants was possible with the initial TLR-activation of MSC versus non-activated MSC or antibiotics alone. Administration of ACT in dogs with naturally occurring musculoskeletal infections involving osseous structures and soft tissues[23] and more recently in a case-controlled study modeling multidrug-resistant MRSA septic arthritis in horses[10] resulted in enhanced bacterial clearance, reduction of pro-inflammatory cytokines, and reduced pain scores compared to antibiotic treatment alone. These findings indicate that pre-conditioning of MSC with immune adjuvants or immunomodulatory substances may be an effective to enhance bacterial clearance even in the face of multiple drug resistances and studies are ongoing to further investigate optimal route(s) of administration, timing of injections, cell source and methods for slow delivery via medical devices or scaffolds to reduce the need for repeated injections.

FUTURE DIRECTIONS WITH MICROCAPSULES AND EXOSOME-BASED THERAPIES

Recent efforts have focused on the development of methods to deliver bioactive factors secreted by MSCs that are integral to the treatment of infection and stimulation of tissue healing while avoiding the legislative constraints associated with the injection of cellular products.[4,24–34] If the observed therapeutic effects of MSCs can be maintained, "cell-free" MSC therapies may offer several advantages, including reduced risk of immune recognition and induction of inflammation due to allograft-associated immune rejection or tumor formation at the site of injected or engrafted cells.[35–38] Efforts to date have involved the packaging of MSC conditioned media, lyophilization and concentration of conditioned media or isolation of extracellular vesicles secreted by MSCs through various techniques.[4,24–34]

Conditioned media from human and equine MSC has demonstrated potential to improve cutaneous wound healing which may be of relevance in the treatment of infection as well.[3,39,40] Bussche and colleagues[4] investigated the microencapsulation of MSC, a process that involves the immobilization of cells within a polymeric semi-permeable membrane. The method of processing purportedly provides a microenvironment in which MSC, or other cells may proliferate and release bioactive factors while not being subject to potentially toxic external environment conditions.[41,42] Bussche and colleagues[4] demonstrated that equine could be successfully packaged in core-shell hydrogel microcapsules, remained viable during long-term encapsulation, and retained MSC characteristics, and that these cells, following encapsulation, induced similar efficacy as non-encapsulated MSCs in their ability to induce migration and gene expression of responder cells (eg, dermal fibroblasts), which may indicate therapeutic potential in wound healing.

Extracellular vesicles (EVs) from multiple cell sources including MSC have gained recent attention as messengers in intercellular communication through the transfer of proteins, lipids, and RNAs in multiple physiological processes.[43] EVs are broadly categorized into three subgroups based on size and biogenesis to include 1) exosomes (40–150 nm) that are released extracellularly when multivesicular bodies fuse with the cell membrane, 2) microvesicles (150–1000 nm) derived from budding of the plasma membrane, and 3) apoptotic bodies (50–2000 nm).[43] Due to their small size, exosome and microvesicle based therapies offer several therapeutic advantages over use of whole MSC as a potential cell-free therapy to minimize side effects such as pulmonary embolism and regulatory concerns raised previously.[43]

In this context of treatment of infection, EVs released from MSCs have been demonstrated to retain antimicrobial characteristics.[44] Multiple previous studies have investigated the implementation of EVs in the context of diseases related to inflammation[43] and to treat various infectious disorders from sepsis to diabetic wound healing to mastitis in dairy cows.[45–50] In the treatment of joint disease, which may be relevant to equine practitioners in the context of treating septic arthritis, MSC-EVs from MSCs stimulated with TGF-ß and IFN-γ have been shown to suppress T-cell proliferation and induce T-reg transformation,[51] to inhibit adverse effects of inflammation on chondrocytes *in vitro* through the abrogation of pro-inflammatory interleukins and TNF-α upregulation of COX-2 pathways and collagenase activity,[52] and to promote cartilage regeneration in a rat model of osteochondral defect *in vivo*,[53] as well as enhanced intrinsic healing in multiple animal models of orthopedic disease including rotator cuff and Achilles tendon repair when incorporated into scaffolds or hydrogels.[54–58] Several groups have recently demonstrated EV isolation from multiple equine derived tissues (bone marrow, endometrium, adipose, amnion), which have largely focused on the effects of EV on joint-derived tissues such as chondrocytes and collagen accumulation.[24–34] While studies examining the biodistribution of EVs in animal models are limited, systemically administered EVs distributed initially quickly to the lungs, spleen, and liver within 30 minutes of injection and then were eliminated through renal and hepatic processing within 6 hours of administration.[59] Further investigation of the incorporation of equine EVs in hydrogels or scaffolds and evaluation of duration of effect and pharmacokinetics of EV when administered locally (eg, intrasynovially) is indicated.

POTENTIAL APPLICATIONS AND CHALLENGES WITH MESENCHYMAL STROMAL CELLS IN EQUINE PRACTICE

Although further case-controlled studies and clinical trials are indicated, based on preliminary evidence, MSC therapy represents a promising potential strategy to improve outcomes in multiple conditions complicated by multi-drug resistant bacterial infections that are commonly treated in equine practice, including septic arthritis.[10] and distal limb wounds.[3] Furthermore, based on evidence for an additive or synergistic effect in reducing quantitative bacterial counts both *in vitro* and *in vivo* when co-administered with antibiotics, extrapolation to additional conditions for which equine patients are presented for treatment including postoperative incisional infection, peritonitis, and pneumonia seem likely as future avenues for this mode of treatment. Immediate administration at the time of presentation presents a clinical challenge due to the length of time necessary to generate autologous cultured cells and potential for reduced quality of cultured products due to donor morbidity in diseased states. However, these challenges may be overcome with the further development of allogeneic or exosome-based strategies pending the navigation of regulatory and manufacturing considerations.

EVIDENCE FOR ANTIMICROBIAL PROPERTIES OF EQUINE PLATELET PRODUCTS

Platelet-rich plasma (PRP) products are used extensively in equine practice for the treatment of musculoskeletal injuries and wounds and have been critically reviewed.[60] These products are believed to promote tissue healing by concentrating and releasing large quantities of growth and chemotactic factors contained within platelet alpha granules at the injury site,[60,61] but both experimental and clinical results have been muddied by PRP preparation variability and lack of a standard equine PRP classification system.[60] More recently, PRP products have been investigated for their additional antimicrobial and immunomodulatory properties.[62,63] These properties stem from the platelet's ability to recognize bacterial pattern associated molecular patterns (PAMPs) via toll-like receptors (TLRs) which activate the platelet to degranulate and release factors such as antimicrobial peptides.[64–69] Antimicrobial peptides are directly antibacterial and maintain this activity against both planktonic and biofilm bacterial phenotypes.[70–72] In addition, antimicrobial peptides can exert potent immunomodulatory and anti-inflammatory effects.[73–76] Antimicrobial peptides have been shown to aid in the functionality of macrophages and neutrophils by increasing their ability to produce reactive intermediates such as superoxide and nitric oxide.[63,65,69,77,78]

Several studies have investigated the general antimicrobial capacity of PRP *in vitro*, observing both bacteriostatic and bactericidal properties.[68,79–87] In addition, PRP can be active against bacteria within biofilms *in vitro*.[67,79–83] *In vivo*, PRP alone or in combination with conventional antimicrobials has shown efficacy in animal models of osteomyelitis, spinal implant infections, and infected surgical wounds.[81,84,88] Platelets can be antibacterial in the absence of plasma[67,69]; however, the addition of plasma can boost the antibacterial capacity of platelets making PRP a superior antibacterial.[89,90] Importantly, activation or lysis of the platelets within PRP can further increase the antibacterial activity of the product by rapidly and thoroughly releasing stores of antimicrobial peptides and other platelet-derived bioactive factors from the platelet alpha granules.[67,79,90]

METHODS TO ENHANCE ANTIMICROBIAL PROPERTIES OF EQUINE PLATELET PRODUCTS

Unlike traditional PRP preparations generated from autologous blood, equine platelet lysate products being investigated for antimicrobial use are generally allogeneic and pooled from multiple donors for several reasons.[90–92] Lysis of platelets both releases antimicrobial peptides as discussed above and renders the product acellular.[67,79,90] It is well known that there is tremendous variability in platelet-derived products based on factors including donor age and gender as well as donor systemic health and hydration status in addition to medications being taken and even time of the blood draw due to the effect of the circadian rhythm on platelet function.[60,93–97] Pooling of platelet lysate from multiple donors reduces such variability and potentially even capitalizes on naturally occurring variability in antimicrobial peptides between donors to generate an optimal end product.[90–92,98] The acellular nature of platelet lysate products is not only critical for the safety of allogeneic pooled use, but could also mitigate the ability of bacteria to exploit intact platelets as a virulence factor.[99]

Several groups have been working to refine equine pooled platelet lysate manufacturing techniques and have demonstrated the efficacy of these products against both gram-positive and gram-negative bacteria *in vitro*[90,91] and against *S. aureus* biofilms *in vivo.*[92] The use of an equine pooled platelet lysate product manufactured via plateletpheresis was initially described as a serum substitute for cell culture,[98] but more recently has been shown to have antimicrobial efficacy against multiple bacterial strains *in vitro* including *S. aureus, E. faecalis*, *E. coli*, and *P. aeruginosa* when cultured in Brain Heart infusion broth.[91] Interestingly, specific effects of the pooled platelet lysate product in this study were unique to each bacterial strain in terms of platelet concentration and lag time after treatment.[91]

The use of an equine pooled platelet lysate product manufactured via fractionation of 50x PRP-lysate enriched for cationic, <10 kDa peptides (termed BIO-PLY for the BIOactive fraction of Platelet-rich plasma LYsate) has also been described and investigated specifically for its efficacy against synovial fluid biofilms.[90,92] BIO-PLY demonstrated anti-biofilm properties and restored traditional antimicrobial efficacy against *S. aureus, S. zooepidemicus, P. aeruginosa,* and *E. coli* clinical isolates cultured in equine synovial fluid *in vitro.*[90] In an equine septic arthritis model *in vivo,* BIO-PLY combined with the traditional antimicrobial amikacin was able to clear *S. aureus* biofilms while mitigating cartilage degeneration and joint inflammation compared to amikacin alone.[92] Notably, treatment with BIO-PLY and amikacin demonstrated immunomodulatory properties with significant shifts in cytokine responses pertaining particularly to macrophage phenotypes and significantly reduced the loss of infection-associated cartilage proteoglycan content in articular cartilage and decreased synovial tissue fibrosis and inflammation compared to treatment with amikacin alone.[92] These findings are promising for the potential prevention of performance limiting osteoarthritis and persistent pain following joint sepsis.

POTENTIAL APPLICATIONS AND CHALLENGES WITH PLATELET LYSATE PRODUCTS IN EQUINE PRACTICE

As discussed above for MSCs, clinical trials for platelet lysate products are also indicated for a variety of clinical conditions involving biofilm-based infections prior to widespread clinical use. A major advantage to the use of pooled platelet lysate products for the treatment of such infections is their "off-the-shelf" availability for immediate therapy due to the allogeneic and acellular nature of these products. Despite being acellular, caution must still be taken however to ensure lack of immunogenicity as well as to prevent transmission of infectious diseases such as Equine Infectious Anemia (EIA) and Equine Parvovirus-Hepatitis.[100] During the manufacturing process, immunoglobulins, F(ab) fragments, and major histocompatibility complex (MHC) peptides must be excluded or removed. In addition, all donor horses must be routinely screened for transmissible diseases as defined by USDA APHIS Center for Veterinary Biologics.

SUMMARY

In summary, increased recognition of the prevalence of antibiotic resistance and biofilm-based infections in clinical practice has prompted the evaluation of alternative antimicrobial treatments, including regenerative and biologic therapies such as MSC and platelet products. While initial *in vitro* and *in vivo* data, as well as case-controlled studies in veterinary species, indicate efficacy, including in the face of bacterial biofilms as would be the case in septic arthritis, current challenges include compliance with regulations from governing bodies regarding the use of cell-based products and allogeneic products as well as practicality of administration at the time of presentation if autologous cell-based products are implemented. Future directions of this field may focus on exosome-based or lyophilized versions of MSCs and the lysate version of platelet products to overcome these hurdles in the face of mounting pressure from antibiotic-resistant organisms in practice. Combined use of MSCs and platelet lysate products should also be considered and is just starting to be explored.

CLINICS CARE POINTS

- Application of biologic therapies including MSC and platelet lysate products may improve outcomes in multiple conditions complicated by multi-drug resistant bacterial infections and biofilms treated in equine practice, including septic arthritis and distal limb wounds.
- Co-administration of MSC or platelet products with antibiotics is indicated due to an additive or synergistic effect in reducing bacterial counts when administered in conjunction.
- Further development of allogeneic or exosome based MSC strategies may reduce clinical challenges in administration of MSC at time of presentation pending navigation of regulatory and manufacturing considerations.
- Pooled platelet lysate products represent an option for 'off-the-shelf' availability for immediate therapy due to their allogeneic and acellular nature.

CONFLICTS OF INTEREST

Authors S.W. Dow, L.M. Pezzanite, L. Chow and L.R. Goodrich declare that a patent application has been filed covering the antimicrobial cellular therapy technology described here. L.M. Pezzanite reports that she holds stock options in eQCell Inc. SWD reports that he holds stock options in eQCell Inc. L.R. Goodrich reports that she holds stock options in eQCell and Advanced Regenerative Therapies. Authors J.M. Gilbertie and L.V. Schnabel declare that a patent application has been filed for the BIO-PLY technology described here.

REFERENCES

1. Smith RKW. Mesenchymal stem cell therapy for equine tendinopathy. Disability Rehab 2008;30:1752–8.
2. Cortes-Araya Y, Amilon K, Rink B, et al. Comparison of antibacterial and immunological properties of mesenchymal stem/stromal cells from equine bone marrow, endometrium, and adipose tissue. Stem Cells Dev 2018;27:1518–25.
3. Harman R, Yang S, He M, et al. Antimicrobial peptides secreted by equine mesenchymal stromal cells inhibit the growth of bacteria commonly found in skin wounds. Stem Cell Res Ther 2017;8:157.

4. Bussche L, Harman RM, Syracuse BA, et al. Microencapsulated equine mesenchymal stromal cells promote cutaneous wound healing *in vitro*. Stem Cell Res Ther 2015;6:66.
5. MacDonald ES, Barrett JG. The potential of mesenchymal stem cells to treat systemic inflammation in horses. Front Vet Sci 2020;6:507.
6. Sherman AB, Gilger BC, Berglund AK, et al. Effect of bone marrow-derived mesenchymal stem cells and stem cell supernatant on equine corneal wound healing *in vitro*. Stem Cell Res Ther 2017;8:120.
7. Davis AB, Schnabel LV, Gilger BC. Subconjunctival bone marrow-derived mesenchymal stem cell therapy as a novel treatment alternative for equine immune-mediated keratitis: a case series. Vet Ophthalmol 2019;22:674–82.
8. Ferris DJ, Frisbie DD, Kisiday JD, et al. Clinical outcome after intra-articular administration of bone marrow derived mesenchymal stem cells in 33 horses with stifle injury. Vet Surg 2014;43:255–65.
9. Pezzanite L, Chow L, Johnson V, et al. Toll-like receptor activation of equine mesenchymal stromal cells to enhance antibacterial activity and immunomodulatory cytokine secretion. Vet Surg 2021;50:858–71.
10. Pezzanite LM, Chow L, Phillips J, et al. TLR-activated mesenchymal stromal cell therapy and antibiotics to treat multi-drug resistant Staphylococcal septic arthritis in an equine model. Ann Transl Med 2022;10:1157. https://doi.org/10.21037/atm-22-1746.
11. Russell KA, Garbin LC, Wong JM, et al. Mesenchymal stromal cells as potential antimicrobial for veterinary use – a comprehensive review. Front Microbiol 2020;11:606404.
12. Marx C, Gardner S, Harman RM, et al. The mesenchymal stromal cell secretome impairs methicillin-resistant Staphylococcus aureus biofilms via cysteine protease activity in the equine model. Stem Cells Transl Med 2020;9:746–57.
13. Chow L, Johnson V, Impastato R, et al. Antibacterial activity of human mesenchymal stem cells mediated directly by constitutively secreted factors and indirectly by activation of innate immune effector cells. Stem Cells Transl Med 2020;9:235–49.
14. Pezzanite LM, Chow L, Strumpf A, et al. Immune activated cellular therapy for drug resistant infections: rationale, mechanisms, and implications for veterinary medicine. Vet Sci 2022;9:610.
15. Pezzanite L, Chow L, Griffenhagen G, et al. Impact of three different serum sources on functional properties of equine mesenchymal stromal cells. Front Vet Sci 2021;8:634064.
16. Karnieli O, Friedner OM, Allickson JG, et al. A consensus introduction to serum replacements and serum-free media for cellular therapies. Cytotherapy 2017;19:155–69.
17. European Commission. Note for guidance on minimizing the risk of transmitting animal spongiform enceaphlopathy agents via human and veterinary medicinal products (EMA/410/01 rev.3). Brussels: Official Journal of the European Union; 2011.
18. European Medicines Agency. Guideline on the use of bovine serum in the manufacture of human biological medicinal products 2013. London: European Medicines Agency; 2013.
19. Mendicino M, Bailey AM, Wonnacott K, et al. MSC-based product characterization for clinical trials: an FDA perspective. Cell Stem Cell 2014;14:141–5.

20. Asami T, Ishii M, Namkoong H, et al. Anti-inflammatory roles of mesenchymal stromal cells during acute Streptococcus pneumoniae pulmonary infection in mice. Cytotherapy 2018;20:302–13.
21. Gorskaya YF, Tukhvatulin AI, Nesterenko VG. NNLR2 and TLR3, TLR4, TLR5 ligands, injected in vivo, improve after 1 h the efficiency of cloning and proliferative activity of bone marrow multipotent stromal cells and reduce the content of osteogenic multipotent stromal cells in CBA mice. Microbiol Immunol 2017;163:356–60.
22. Aqdas M, Singh S, Amir M, et al. Cumulative signaling through NOD-2 and TLR-4 eliminates the mycobacterium tuberculosis concealed inside the mesenchymal stem cells. Front Cell Infect Microbiol 2021;11:669168.
23. Johnson V, Webb T, Norman A, et al. Activated mesenchymal stem cells interact with antibiotics and host innate immune responses to control chronic bacterial infections. Sci Rep 2017;7:9575.
24. Kartunnen J, Heiskanen M, Joki T, et al. Effect of cell culture media on extracellular vesicle secretion from mesenchymal stromal cells and neurons. Eur J Cell Biol 2022;101:151270.
25. Tasma Z, Hou W, Damani T, et al. Production of extracellular vesicles from equine embryo-derived mesenchymal stromal cells. Reproduction 2022;164:143–54.
26. Soukup R, Gerner I, Gultekin S, et al. Characterisation of extracellular vesicles from equine mesenchymal stem cells. Int J Mol Sci 2022;23:5858.
27. Contentin R, Jammes M, Bourdon B, et al. Bone marrow MSC secretome increases equine articular chondrocyte collagen accumulation and their migratory capacities. Int J Mol Sci 2022;23:5795.
28. Hotham WE, Thompson C, Szu-Ting L, et al. The anti-inflammatory effects of equine bone marrow stem cell-derived extracellular vesicles on autologous chondrocytes. Vet Rec Open 2021;8:e22.
29. Arevalo-Turrubiarte M, Baratta M, Ponti G, et al. Extracellular vesicles from equine mesenchymal stem cells decrease inflammation markers in chondrocytes in vitro. Equine Vet J 2022;54:1133–43.
30. Navarrete F, Sen Wong Y, Cabezas J, et al. Distinctive cellular transcriptomic signature and microRNA cargo of extracellular vesicles of horse adipose and endometrial mesenchymal stem cells from the same donors. Cell Reprogram 2020;22:311–27.
31. Capomaccio S, Cappelli K, Bazzucchi C, et al. Equine adipose-derived mesenchymal stromal cells release extracellular vesicles enclosing different subsets of small RNAs. Stem Cells Int 2019;4957806. https://doi.org/10.1155/2019/4957806.
32. Boere J, Malda J, van de Lest CHA, et al. Extracellular vesicles in joint disease and therapy. Front Immunol 2018;9:2575.
33. Pascucci L, Dall'Aglio C, Bazzucchi C, et al. Horse adipose-derived mesenchymal stromal cells constitutively produce membrane vesicles: a morphological study. Histol Histopathol 2015;30:549–57.
34. Lange-Consiglio A, Perrini C, Tasquier R, et al. Equine amniotic microvesicles and their anti-inflammatory potential in a tenocyte model in vitro. Stem Cells Dev 2016;25(8):610–21.
35. Haarer J, Johnson CL, Soeder Y, et al. Caveats of mesenchymal stem cell therapy in solid organ transplantation. Transpl Int 2015;28:1–9.
36. Maguire G. Stem cell therapy without the cells. Commun Integr Biol 2013;6:e26631.

37. Pezzanite LM, Fortier LA, Antczak DF, et al. Equine allogeneic bone marrow-derived mesenchymal stromal cells elicit antibody responses *in vivo.* Stem Cell Res Ther 2015;6:54.
38. Berglund AK, Schnabel LV. Allogeneic major histocompatibility complex-mismatched equine bone marrow derived mesenchymal stem cells are targeted for death by cytotoxic anti-major histocompatibility complex antibodies. Equine Vet J 2017;49:539–44.
39. Chen CP, Chen YY, Huang JP, et al. The effect of conditioned medium derived from human placental multipotent mesenchymal stromal cells on neutrophils: possible implications for placental infection. Mol Hum Reprod 2014;20:1117–25.
40. Akram KM, Samad S, Spiteri MA, et al. Mesenchymal stem cells promote alveolar epithelial cell wound repair in vitro through distinct migratory and paracrine mechanisms. Respir Res 2013;14:9.
41. Chang TMS. Therapeutic applications of polymeric artificial cells. Nat Rev Drug Discov 2005;4:221–5.
42. Orive G, Santos E, Pedraz JL, et al. Application of cell encapsulation for controlled delivery of biological therapeutics. Adv Drug Deliv Rev 2014;67. https://doi.org/10.1016/j.addr.2013.07.009. 683-14.
43. Yin K, Wang S, Zhao RC. Exosomes from mesenchymal stem/stromal cells: a new therapeutic paradigm. Biomark Res 2018;7:8.
44. Jimenez-Puerta GJ, Marchal JA, Ruiz EL, et al. Role of mesenchymal stromal cells as therapeutic agents: potential mechanisms of action and implications in their clinical use. J Clin Med 2020;9:445.
45. Ghai S, Saini S, Ansari S, et al. Allogenic umbilical cord blood-mesenchymal stem cells are more effective than antibiotics in alleviating subclinical mastitis in dairy cows. Theriogenology 2022;187:141–51.
46. Geng X, Qi Y, Liu X, et al. A multifunctional antibacterial and self-healing hydrogel laden with bone marrow mesenchymal stem cell-derived exosomes for accelerating diabetic wound healing. Biomater Adv 2022;133:112613.
47. Alikhani H, Shokoohian B, Rezasoltani S, et al. Application of stem cell-derived extracellular vesicles as an innovative theranostics in microbial diseases. Front Microbiol 2021;12:785856.
48. You J, Fu Z, Zou L. Mechanism and potential of extracellular vesicles derived from mesenchymal stem cells for the treatment of infectious diseases. Front Microbiol 2021;12:761338.
49. Marrazzo P, Pizzuti V, Zia S, et al. Microfluidics tools for enhanced characterization of therapeutic stem cells and prediction of their potential antimicrobial secretome. Antibiotics 2021;10:750.
50. Cheng Y, Cao X, Qin L. Mesenchymal stem cell-derived extracellular vesicles: a novel cell-free therapy for sepsis. Front Immunol 2020;11:647.
51. Zhang Q, Fu L, Liang Y, et al. Exosomes originating from MSCs stimulated with TGF-ß and IFN-γ promote T-reg differentiation. J Cell Physiol 2018;233(9):6832–40.
52. Vonik LA, van Dooremalen SFJ, Liv N, et al. Mesenchymal stromal/stem cell-derived extracellular vesicles promote human cartilage regeneration in vitro. Theranostics 2018;8(4):906–20.
53. Zhang S, Chu WC, Lai RC, et al. Exosomes derived from human embryonic mesenchymal stem cells promote osteochondral regeneration. Osteoarthritis Cartilage 2016;24(12):2135–40.

54. Shi G, Lonng Z, De la Vega RE, et al. Purified exosome product enhances chondrocyte survival and regeneration by modulating inflammation and promoting chondrogenesis. Regen Med 2022. https://doi.org/10.2217/rme-2022-0132.
55. Wan R, Hussain A, Behfar A, et al. The therapeutic potential of exosomes in soft tissue repair and regeneration. Int J Mol Sci 2022;23:3869.
56. Wellings EP, Huang TC, Li J, et al. Intrinsic tendon regeneration after application of purified exosome product: an in vivo study. Orthop J Sports Med 2021;9. https://doi.org/10.1177/23259671211062929. 23259671211062929.
57. Ren Y, Zhang S, Wang Y, et al. Effects of purified exosome product on rotator cuff tendon-bone healing in vitro and in vivo. Biomaterials 2021;276:121019.
58. Qi J, Liu Q, Reisdorf RL, et al. Characterization of a purified exosome product and its effects on canine flexor tenocyte biology. J Orthop Res 2020;38: 1845–55.
59. Lai CP, Mardini S, Ericsson M, et al. Dynamic biodistribution of extracellular vesicles in vivo using a multimodal imaging reporter. ACS Nano 2014;8(1):483–94.
60. Camargo Garbin L, Lopez C, Carmona JU. A critical overview of the use of platelet-rich plasma in equine medicine over the last decade. Front Vet Sci 2021;8:641818.
61. Boswell SG, Cole BJ, Sundman EA, et al. Platelet-rich plasma: a milieu of bioactive factors. Arthroscopy 2012;28(3):429–39.
62. Moojen DJF, Everts PAM, Schure RM, et al. Antimicrobial activity of platelet-leukocyte gel against staphylococcus aureus. J Orthop Res 2008;26:404–10.
63. Aktan Í, Dunkel B, Cunningham FM. Equine platelets inhibit E. coli growth and can be activated by bacterial lipopolysaccharide and lipoteichoic acid although superoxide anion production does not occur and platelet activation is not associated with enhanced production by neutrophils. Vet Immunol Immunopathol 2013;152:209–17.
64. Cox D, Kerrigan SW, Watson SP. Platelets and the innate immune system: Mechanisms of bacterial-induced platelet activation. J Thromb Haemostasis 2011;9: 1097–107.
65. Morrell CN, Aggrey AA, Chapman LM, et al. Emerging roles for platelets as immune and inflammatory cells. Blood 2014;123:2759–67.
66. Garraud O, Hamzeh-Cognasse H, Pozzetto B, et al. Bench-to-bedside review: Platelets and active immune functions - new clues for immunopathology? Crit Care 2013;17:236.
67. Tang Y-Q, Yeaman MR, Selsted ME. Antimicrobial peptides from human platelets. Infect Immun 2002;70:6524–33.
68. Tohidnezhad M, Varoga D, Wruck CJ, et al. Platelets display potent antimicrobial activity and release human beta-defensin 2. Platelets 2012;23:217–23.
69. Kraemer BF, Campbell RA, Schwertz H, et al. Novel anti-bacterial activities of β-defensin 1 in human platelets: Suppression of pathogen growth and signaling of neutrophil extracellular trap formation. PLoS Pathog 2011;7:e1002355.
70. Reffuveille F, De La Fuente-Nunez C, Mansour S, et al. A broad-spectrum anti-biofilm peptide enhances antibiotic action against bacterial biofilms. Antimicrobial Agents Chemother 2014;58:5363–71.
71. Pletzer D, Hancock REWW. Antibiofilm peptides: Potential as broadspectrum agents. J Bacteriol 2016;198:2572–8.
72. De La Fuente-Núñez C, Cardoso MH, De Souza Cândido E, et al. Synthetic antibiofilm peptides. Biochimica et Biophysica Acta - Biomembranes 2016;1858: 1061–9.

73. Mansour SC, de la Fuente-Núñez C, Hancock REWW. Peptide IDR-1018: Modulating the immune system and targeting bacterial biofilms to treat antibiotic-resistant bacterial infections. J Pept Sci 2015;21:323–9.
74. Nijnik A, Madera L, Ma S, et al. Synthetic cationic peptide IDR-1002 provides protection against bacterial infections through chemokine induction and enhanced leukocyte recruitment. J Immunol 2010;184:2539–50.
75. Niyonsaba F, Madera L, Afacan N, et al. The innate defense regulator peptides IDR-HH2, IDR-1002, and IDR-1018 modulate human neutrophil functions. J Leukoc Biol 2013;94:159–70.
76. Torres-Juarez F, Cardenas-Vargas A, Montoya-Rosales A, et al. LL-37 immunomodulatory activity during Mycobacterium tuberculosis infection in macrophages. Infect Immun 2015;83:4495–503.
77. Muehlmann LA, Michelotto PV, Nunes EA, et al. PAF increases phagocytic capacity and superoxide anion production in equine alveolar macrophages and blood neutrophils. Res Vet Sci 2012;93:393–7.
78. Speth C, Löffler J, Krappmann S, et al. Platelets as immune cells in infectious diseases. Future Microbiol 2013;8:1431–51.
79. Burnouf T, Chou ML, Wu YW, et al. Antimicrobial activity of platelet (PLT)-poor plasma, PLT-rich plasma, PLT gel, and solvent/detergent-treated PLT lysate biomaterials against wound bacteria. Transfusion 2013;53:138–46.
80. Bielecki TM, Gazdzik TS, Arendt J, et al. Antibacterial effect of autologous platelet gel enriched with growth factors and other active substances: an in vitro study. Journal of Bone and Joint Surgery - British 2007;89-B:417–20.
81. Li GY, Yin JM, Ding H, et al. Efficacy of leukocyte- and platelet-rich plasma gel (L-PRP gel) in treating osteomyelitis in a rabbit model. J Orthop Res 2013;31: 949–56.
82. Mariani E, Filardo G, Canella V, et al. Platelet-rich plasma affects bacterial growth in vitro. Cytotherapy 2014;16:1294–304.
83. Intravia J, Allen DA, Durant TJ, et al. In vitro evaluation of the anti-bacterial effect of two preparations of platelet rich plasma compared with cefazolin and whole blood. Muscles, Ligaments and Tendons Journal 2014;4:79–84.
84. Li H, Hamza T, Tidwell JE, et al. Unique antimicrobial effects of platelet-rich plasma and its efficacy as a prophylaxis to prevent implant-associated spinal infection. Advanced Healthcare Materials 2013;2:1277–84.
85. Drago L, Bortolin M, Vassena C, et al. Antimicrobial activity of pure platelet-rich plasma against microorganisms isolated from oral cavity. BMC Microbiol 2013; 13:47.
86. López C, Carmona JU, Giraldo CE, et al. Bacteriostatic effect of equine pure platelet-rich plasma and other blood products against methicillin-sensitive Staphylococcus aureus. An in vitro study. Vet Comp Orthop Traumatol 2014; 27(5):372–8.
87. López C, Alvarez ME, Carmona JU. Temporal bacteriostatic effect and growth factor loss in equine platelet components and plasma cultured with methicillin-sensitive and methicillin-resistant staphylococcus aureus: a comparative in vitro study. Vet Med Int 2014;525826. https://doi.org/10.1155/2014/525826.
88. Cetinkaya RA, Yilmaz S, Ünlü A, et al. The efficacy of platelet-rich plasma gel in MRSA-related surgical wound infection treatment: an experimental study in an animal model. Eur J Trauma Emerg Surg 2018;44:859–67.

89. Drago L, Bortolin M, Vassena C, et al. Plasma components and platelet activation are essential for the antimicrobial properties of autologous platelet-rich plasma: an in vitrostudy. PLoS One 2014;9:e107813.
90. Gilbertie JM, Schaer TP, Schubert AG, et al. Platelet-rich plasma lysate displays antibiofilm properties and restores antimicrobial activity against synovial fluid biofilms in vitro. J Orthop Res 2020;38:1365–74.
91. Gordon J, Álvarez-Narváez S, Peroni JF. Antimicrobial effects of equine platelet lysate. Front Vet Sci 2021;19:703414.
92. Gilbertie JM, Schaer TP, Engiles JB, et al. A platelet-rich plasma-derived biologic clears staphylococcus aureus biofilms while mitigating cartilage degeneration and joint inflammation in a clinically relevant large animal infectious arthritis model. Front Cell Infect Microbiol 2022;30:895022.
93. Giraldo CE, López C, Álvarez ME, et al. Effects of the breed, sex and age on cellular content and growth factor release from equine pure-platelet rich plasma and pure-platelet rich gel. BMC Vet Res 2013;12:29.
94. Xiong G, Lingampalli N, Koltsov JCB, et al. Men and Women Differ in the Biochemical Composition of Platelet-Rich Plasma. Am J Sports Med 2018;46:409–19.
95. Rinnovati R, Romagnoli N, Gentilini F, et al. The influence of environmental variables on platelet concentration in horse platelet-rich plasma. Acta Vet Scand 2016;4. https://doi.org/10.1186/s13028-016-0226-3. 58:45.
96. Gilbertie JM, Davis JL, Davidson GS, et al. Oral reserpine administration in horses results in low plasma concentrations that alter platelet biology. Equine Vet J 2019;51:537–43.
97. Scheer FA, Michelson AD, Frelinger AL 3rd, et al. The human endogenous circadian system causes greatest platelet activation during the biological morning independent of behaviors. PLoS One 2011;6:e24549.
98. Naskou MC, Norton NA, Copland IB, et al. Innate immune responses of equine monocytes cultured in equine platelet lysate. Vet Immunol Immunopatholol 2018;195:65–71.
99. Liesenborghs L, Verhamme P, Vanassche T. Staphylococcus aureus, master manipulator of the human hemostatic system. J Thromb Haemostasis 2018;16:441–54.
100. Tomlinson JE, Kapoor A, Kumar A, et al. Viral testing of 18 consecutive cases of equine serum hepatitis: a prospective study (2014-2018). J Vet Intern Med 2019;33:251–7.

Printed and bound by CPI Group (UK) Ltd, Croydon, CR0 4YY
03/10/2024
01040477-0012